RUNNING YOUR FIRST MARATHON

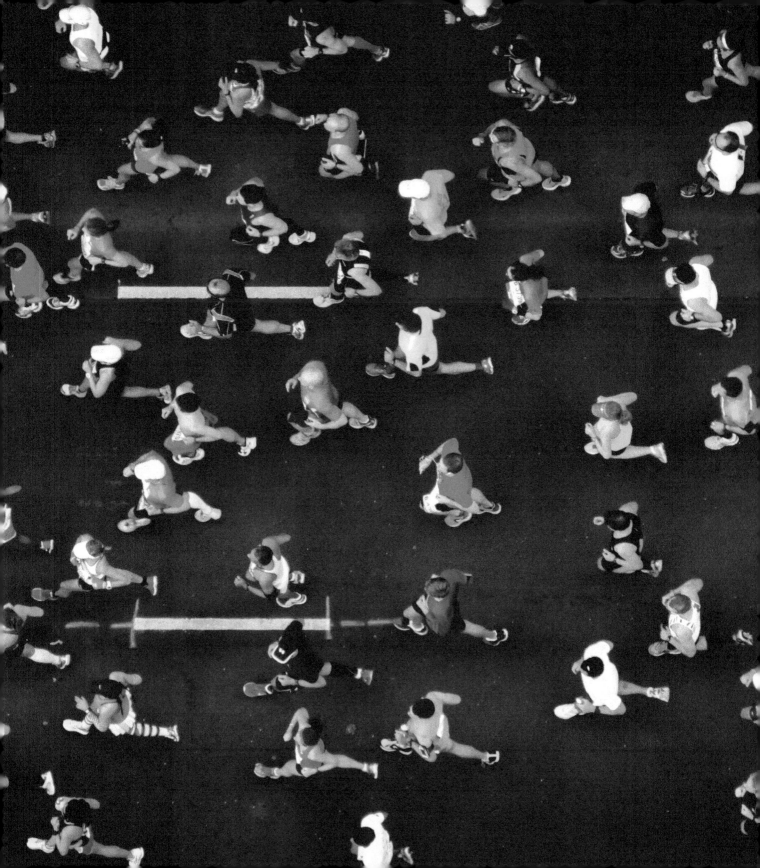

RUNNING YOUR FIRST

MARATHON

THE COMPLETE 20-WEEK

MARATHON TRAINING PLAN

Andrew Kastor

ROCKRIDGE
PRESS

In memory of Gabe Proctor.
Your effortless stride was a pleasure to watch.
I'll always remember our friendship.
Rest in peace, Champ.

CONTENTS

INTRODUCTION

"The will to win is nothing without the will to prepare."

—Juma Ikangaa, 1989 New York City Marathon Winner

n November 2001, less than two months after the September 11 attack on the World Trade Center, I had the great privilege of running in the New York City Marathon, and it was by far my most memorable race to date. As a former competitive runner, I didn't finish as fast as I would have liked (in fact, I basically bonked), but the combination of it being my first marathon and the emotions I, and everyone else on the course, felt running 26.2 miles through that strong, beautiful, resilient city more than made up for my slightly disappointing finish time. It was then that I realized there are many amazing reasons why people run this distance.

For months, I had visualized running straight through the five boroughs that make up the NYC Marathon course at a pace of 6:52 per mile, with a projected three-hour finish time. I had prepared meticulously . . . or so I thought. I started off strong. I had the unique opportunity to line up directly behind the elite women, as my girlfriend at the time (now wife), Deena, was competing in the women's professional field (it was her first marathon, too). And at 10 a.m. a cannon rang out a thunderous boom, signaling to me and the 30,000 other athletes patiently waiting at the base of the Verrazano-Narrows Bridge that it was time for us to climb out of Staten Island and begin our long 26.2-mile journey up to Central Park.

Unfortunately, the race didn't go as planned, and I was walking by mile 20. In classic runners' speak, "I hit the wall" (or "my wheels came off," or "I bonked"). Afterward, I asked myself a series of questions: Why did this morning go so poorly? Did I train correctly? Was my pacing too aggressive? Was it something I ate . . . or didn't eat? I finally realized that the answers to all of these questions (and more) led to me being underprepared and ultimately not reaching my goal.

As a coach to all different types of runners, from first-time 5Kers to Olympic marathoners, over the last 21 years, it has been my job to try to prevent others from making the same kinds of mistakes. The first coaching position I landed was for a distance-running program with seven athletes on a community college track team in Southern California. Six years later, I started a nonprofit running club in Mammoth Lakes, California, called the High Sierra Striders, which consisted of athletes of all abilities and ages whose biggest motivation to run was "to slow the rate of inevitable decline," as one older gentleman graciously put it. Then in 2012, I was hired on as the coaching director for the Los Angeles Marathon and the LA Road Runners, a group of a thousand beginner to advanced runners who do strategically prescribed training runs together every Saturday morning. Today, I coach the Mammoth Track Club, a team that prepares elite athletes for national, world, and Olympic championship competitions.

I've personally completed four marathons, and I make a point to draw from my own experience, as well as my passion for and knowledge of running, every time I create a training plan for someone else. I've worked with athletes who simply want to finish a marathon and those who want to finish faster than ever before. Regardless of their goals and abilities, every single one of them has learned to overcome some of the physical and mental rigors of marathon training. So it is my firm belief that with the proper guidance, anyone can find the sport of marathon running to be immensely rewarding.

That's where this book comes in. I will discuss everything you need to know when preparing for and attempting to finish your first marathon—tips on choosing the right race, training advice (and plans) to help you reach your goals, ways to select the proper gear, suggestions of what to eat and drink during all those long runs, dynamic warm-ups and stretches you can do to reduce your risk of injury and improve your performance, ideas for staying motivated, and much, much more.

My goal as a coach is to give you all the information you need to make it to the starting line healthy and the finish line happy.

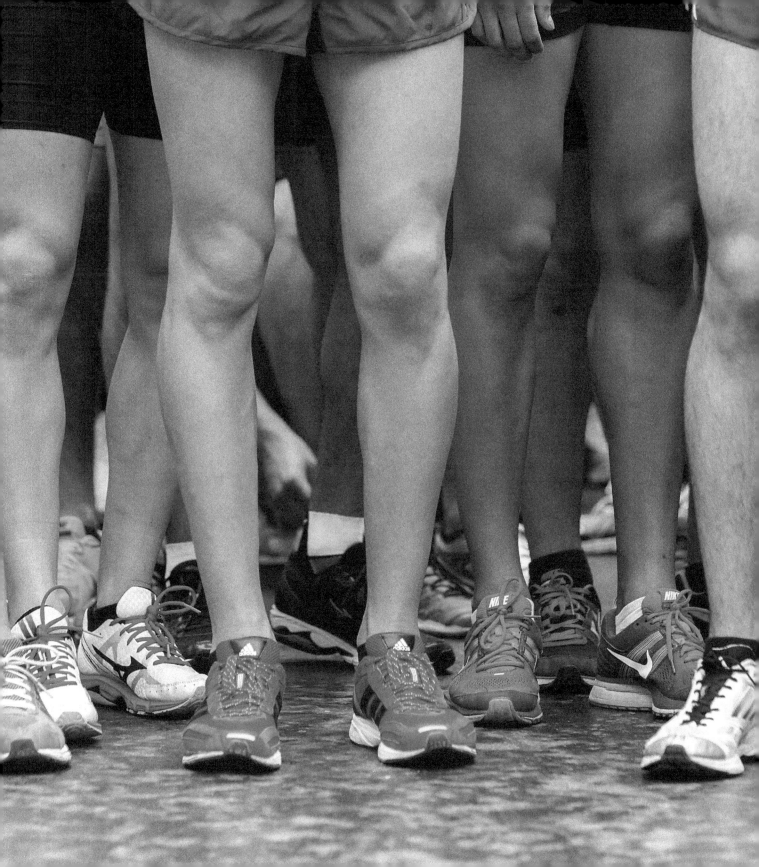

1

THE STARTING LINE

Running a marathon is a daunting task. History has it that the actual distance was determined in commemoration of the run that Greek soldier Pheidippides completed in 490 BC, from a battlefield near the town of Marathon, Greece, to Athens, to personally announce victory over the Persians. It wasn't until 1896, when the first modern Olympic Games took place in Athens, that the marathon was officially introduced as a sanctioned event, and it is still the longest distance running event in both the Olympics and the World Track and Field Championships.

It's human nature to want to conquer a challenge. "Because it's there," as the incomparable George Mallory famously said about climbing Mount Everest back in the 1920s. Completing a marathon is basically the modern-day weekend warrior's version of Mt. Everest. And interest in marathons continues to grow in the United States; RunningUSA.org notes that there are 1,100 races to choose from, and just over half a million runners finishing a marathon here every year since 2010.

Regardless of what brings you to the starting line—a personal challenge, weight loss, competing for an age-group medal, peer pressure from your runner friends, raising money for an important cause—you must dedicate time and energy to your training to mentally and physically prepare yourself for the distance.

SETTING EXPECTATIONS

Ever since I was a freshman in high school, I've dedicated my life to the sport I love, running. I've trained as both a competitor and as a coach, working countless times to get myself and other athletes across the finish line. I understand the internal drive to challenge one's physical and mental capabilities, and doing a marathon does just that. It takes a substantial amount of work, dedication, commitment, and ambition to complete the journey. It's my intention, in writing this book, to make the process fun and informative for you, whether you're an experienced runner at shorter distance races (5Ks, 10Ks, or half marathons) or you're literally just starting out in the running game. Either way, I understand where you're coming from and will guide you to reaching your goals.

This easy-to-follow guide to marathon training will improve your current fitness level and help you navigate the winding, sometimes hilly, road to the starting line—and eventually, finish line—with confidence, strength, and fun.

But before you begin, I want you to spend a minute to reflect on what your motives are: Did a friend ask you to run a marathon with him or her? Are you running for a charity, raising money for cancer research? Did you decide to tackle 26.2 miles because that's the next logical challenge after running a few half-marathons? Whatever your motivations are, hold them tightly to your chest. You'll need to revisit these often during the course of your training, especially when the workouts become tough or you have to wake up at 4 a.m. to squeeze in a run. So, why are you running a marathon? If you're running to achieve your fastest race ever, then this is probably not the book for you. My goal as your coach is to simply get you from start to finish—to help you successfully (and happily) complete your first full marathon.

During the 20-week marathon-training plan, you will be testing your physical and mental abilities harder than ever before. To complete everything outlined in this book, you will need to start thinking and planning ahead.

All athletes need a strategy and a plan to get from point A to point B. Runners who follow a good training plan make changes incrementally, as they are guided to adapt ever so slightly over a period of time, using slow and steady progress to prepare for race day. Without stress, there is no adaptation, no progress. The marathon-training plan I've designed for you will systematically place small doses of stress in the forms of specific types of training runs—long, easy, fast—into your routine, throughout your 20-week training period, to help you build the endurance and strength needed to accomplish your ultimate goal.

The marathon-training plan will strategically help you build speed, endurance, and mental strength. It will also focus on recovery, the periods in between your tough training sessions, in which your mind and muscles need to rest and rebuild with nutrition, sleep, and stretching. Since a runner's body is continuously breaking down, you need proper fuel (diet) and recovery to promote fitness gains and prevent injuries. I will suggest what to do each day of the week and how far and fast to run, so all you have to do is follow along.

By the end of the training plan, right before race day, you'll have logged approximately 700 miles (seriously!), developed the physical and mental strength necessary to complete a marathon, and learned to piece all the different aspects of training together for one big final test of endurance.

CHOOSING AND QUALIFYING FOR YOUR RACE

As a coach, I encourage all of my clients, even professional athletes, to start planning well in advance for their marathons. It is an essential part of the process. Selecting and signing up for a marathon race early, five to six months ahead of time, will set a first-time marathoner up for success, giving you time to slowly build toward your peak goal. Allowing for a slow development of fitness will minimize the risk of injury. Plus, race organizers usually reward those who sign up early with discounted entry fees, so you'll save a few bucks, too.

Most runners like to have a clear goal to aim for, and signing up for a marathon early helps keep the emphasis of the season well defined and cultivates patience, something all marathon runners should possess. It is that patience and control, after all, that will teach you to hold back in the early part of your training and racing and put you in a much stronger position for the second half of your season and race.

Things to Consider Before Signing Up

Doing your homework is essential if you want to choose a marathon that's right for you. I know that some runners can find the race selection process to be a bit overwhelming, so to make it easier (and more enjoyable), I've listed some important factors to consider before you sign up.

Timing. When does the event take place? Selecting a marathon with enough lead-up time is essential for proper training and preparation. A majority of the races are in the fall and spring. Choose one that is about five to six months out, so you have time to prepare for and execute your 20-week training plan. If you opt for a fall marathon, this means you'll be training through summer, which can be hot and challenging at times, depending on where you live. Alternatively, if you go with a spring race . . . yep, you guessed it, you'll be training through the winter, when the days are typically shorter, darker, and colder. Popular races sell out quickly, so don't procrastinate with the registration process. Once you know what you want to sign up for, find out what that entails. For bigger events, there is often a lottery registration system involved, which means that more runners than the race allows apply, and they all get placed on a waiting list. So if you sign up for a lottery, it's also a good idea to choose a backup race, just in case your name doesn't get selected.

Location. Where is it? I always like to choose a marathon that is easily accessible and convenient to get to. Three of the four marathons I've run have been in California, an easy drive from my home in the center of the state. But sometimes it's fun

Great Races for First-Time Marathoners

During my first marathon, in New York City, I went to the starting line with a new friend, Rich Kenah. Rich was a professional 800-meter runner and earned a bronze medal in the 1993 World Indoor Championships for the United States. He had been training for the marathon for a few months and gave me a useful piece of advice just minutes before the race began. He leaned over and said, "Today is just another long run with 30,000 new friends." His memorable comment came at the perfect time. It took a little pressure off and reminded me that this was in fact not a race, but rather an event containing thousands of individual stories, from a bunch of people with the same goal: to cross the notorious finish line in Central Park. As I've traveled around the world, experiencing different marathons, I'm always intrigued to hear about them from the perspective of other runners.

If you plan to only run just one marathon in your life, to simply check off that box on your bucket list, then I encourage you to go big and run a well-known, participant-pleasing marathon to keep you motivated and smiling over the miles. The Rock 'n' Roll race series, for example, offers marathons in places around the globe and is a great way to experience running through a major city. They offer live music with bands at every mile along the course to help keep you moving and focused on the "fun" aspect of the sport.

United States

LOS ANGELES MARATHON, CALIFORNIA
(third Sunday in March)
In 2011, the Los Angeles Marathon introduced its now iconic Stadium-to-the-Sea course (Dodger Stadium to Santa Monica Beach). This rolling course is a brilliant tour of the warm Southern California city.

CHICAGO MARATHON, ILLINOIS
(second Sunday in October)
Speed alert! This marathon is home to many American and world records, thanks to its lightning-fast course that loops through the city and starts and finishes in Grant Park. It typically has great weather conditions, too, making Chicago an easy choice for a big-city marathon experience.

NEW YORK CITY MARATHON, NEW YORK

(first Sunday in November)
Two words: *iconic experience*. There is no other marathon in the world like this. New York City brings the energy, every single time. There are one million fans cheering so loudly along First Avenue that it will make the hair on the back of your neck stand up for miles. The only negative is that this race has one of the most competitive marathon registration lotteries.

HONOLULU MARATHON, HAWAII

(second Sunday in December)
This tropical event is perfect for those who want to fit a Hawaiian vacation in around their first marathon. The course has a few moderate hills to navigate while it circles around Diamond Head on the island of Oahu.

PHILADELPHIA MARATHON, PENNSYLVANIA

(third Sunday in November)
Another fast-course alert! This race is a great opportunity to run on a flat course with good weather through a beautiful city filled with fun crowds. This marathon competes for athletes with the New York City Marathon every fall, as the neighboring cities host their races around the same time.

International

TOKYO MARATHON, JAPAN

(last Sunday in February)
A true destination event, this race has a course that's designed for fast times with a couple of manageable inclines thrown in. The weather is typically very runner-friendly, with cool, damp temps in the low- to mid-50s.

LONDON MARATHON, UNITED KINGDOM

(third Sunday in April)
Many national and world records have been set on this lightning-fast, pancake-flat course. It's also filled with a ridiculous number of historic landmarks, such as Tower Bridge, the Palace of Westminster, and Big Ben.

OTTAWA MARATHON, CANADA

(fourth Sunday in May)
This race, hosted by our friendly neighbors to the north, has been a staple for US athletes since 1974, with a mostly flat loop course that takes you on a tour of the capital.

BERLIN MARATHON, GERMANY

(fourth Sunday in September)
This just might be the fastest course on the planet, home to the current men's world record. The participants pass through where the Berlin Wall once stood and finish with a run through the historic Brandenburg Gate.

ATHENS MARATHON, GREECE

(second Sunday in November)
If you want to go straight to the source, well, this hilly course is where it all started.

to travel (and run) somewhere new. Many runners choose a "destination marathon," which is a trip that is part work and part play. There are even guided marathon touring organizations out there that take runners to all corners of the globe. Ask yourself, "What type of conditions do I like to run in?" The answer to that question could help you narrow your search.

Reliability. Is it a well-established race? If you're going to dedicate five to six months of your life to training and preparing for a race, then selecting one that's well known or well established is always a good idea. This is one way to remove the "what if" factor, and you can rest assured that race organizers will be prepared for you and everyone else come the morning of the race. Races usually need a few iterations to work out the kinks and allow a smooth ride to the finish line, so brand-new, or "first annual," marathons are generally not a great choice, especially if it's your first race.

Route. What does the course look like? Is it flat? Hilly? Does it go through a city with lots of crowd support? Or send you somewhere scenic, where you'll be alone with your thoughts for most of the race? Is it multiple loops of the same short course or one long out-and-back? All of these notes are important to consider when choosing your race. They will also help dictate your training. Ideally, the route will be relatively flat, or not too difficult, and have inspiring scenery.

Cost. How expensive will this race (and whole experience) be? Do you have any budget constraints? If so, take them into account before you sign up. Accommodations, airfare, a rental car, and registration fees can add up very fast. Keep in mind that you'll be burning through a few pairs of running shoes as well (approximately one new pair every 300 miles), which is another cost to factor in. One idea you might want to consider is running the marathon for a charity, which means you'll have to raise a certain amount of money for a good cause, but registration fees are often waived as a result.

Most marathons are beginner friendly, meaning that the only "qualifying standard" is that you commit to finishing under their predetermined cut-off time. In other words, you either finish the race at a certain pace (for example, the Los Angeles Marathon has a cut-off time of 6 hours, 30 minutes, and 59 seconds, or running at a pace of 14:54 per mile), or they will close the course and your time will not be officially recorded. So how do you know if you'll be fast enough to cross the finish line? See the appendix (page 133) to extrapolate your predicted marathon finish time from your shorter race times.

There are a few marathons, such as the granddaddy of all races, the Boston Marathon, that have time standards runners must meet to qualify. The Boston Athletic Association (BAA) has tightened their qualification standards over the years due to the increasing popularity of its historic event. To qualify for this marathon, runners must meet time standards set by the BAA based on gender and age. Qualifying times can also be met only on certain BAA-approved courses.

KEEP IN MIND

Here are a few essential things to remember as you start your marathon-training journey.

Etch out time in your daily schedule for training. This can be challenging, but it is so incredibly important. It's also for only five to six months and will make all the difference come race day. Remember, you can basically accomplish anything if you get up early enough!

Get an appropriate pair of shoes for your feet and the type of training you'll be doing. Check out chapter 2 for information on purchasing running shoes.

Grab a partner! Training with a group or friend is typically much more enjoyable. Sharing those miles with someone else is not only a fun experience, but it also adds a level of accountability, since you have to show up to meet others for your workouts. Chapter 7 covers building your support team and connecting with fellow runners.

You're going to be tired! You are asking your body to give all it has to give. The physical and mental demands will inevitably be draining as you'll be pushing it beyond the farthest distance you've ever gone before. You'll need to focus on recovery and plan to sleep an extra 30 to 60 minutes every night.

Proper fueling is essential for performance and recovery. You'll need to commit to eating well every day of training. Fruits and vegetables are essential for repairing damaged muscle (and tendon) tissues. Muscle-building hormones are constantly being depleted, and the best way to replenish those is to eat a well-balanced diet.

Treat yourself to a sports recovery massage a few times during the season . . . if your budget allows for it. This is a great way to lower your risk of injury and boost your recovery. Staying hydrated is also a key component to recovery and preparing your body for daily workouts and training runs. Plan to carry a bottle of water around with you everywhere you go. Sipping water throughout the day is a great way to stay on top of your hydration and keep your body in prime training mode.

Reduce all current sporting activity obligations. Chances are, if you're considering running a marathon, you're a fairly active person and possibly involved in other sports. However, all of your energy should be spent on running and strategic cross-training to help boost your marathon performance (see chapter 5). If you belong to a league, it would be wise to consider hitting the pause button on that while you're in training. The last thing you want is to strain a muscle playing beach volleyball or softball, which could limit your chances of achieving your finish-line goal.

Plan to run one or two other shorter races leading up to your big event. Adding smaller races to your schedule will help keep your motivation high and your training on track.

Keep in mind that you will see highs and lows throughout your training. Things don't always go as planned. Every runner is likely to miss a workout or two due to circumstances that are out of his or her control. Always keep in mind that a race is not won or lost on one single (or a few) workout(s).

Your marathon success depends on the accumulation of training over the 20-week season. Your training and your history as a runner will get you across the finish line.

Remember why you signed up to run a marathon in the first place. Frequently remind yourself of the challenge and the goals you've set for yourself—this will help keep you motivated as you train.

Keep a training log of all of your workouts and miles. Before race day, flip through it all to remind yourself of how hard you've worked over the last five to six months. Know that you have every reason to finish strong and happy.

TIPS FOR SUCCESSFUL TRAINING

Before you start the training plan in this book, get comfortable running 25 to 35 miles per week. This weekly mileage will serve as a solid base of running to build from. If you're not there yet, then work your way up slowly and gradually by adding 5 to 10 minutes to each of your daily runs.

Be patient with your training and the progress. One of the biggest mistakes people make when starting a running program is to go out too quickly in the first couple of weeks. Later in the book, I will talk about the importance of pacing yourself and how to do it successfully (page 35).

Take recovery, or "off," days seriously. This is important to stay healthy and injury-free when training. I usually recommend taking complete "off" days from running or cross-training after very hard or very long training sessions to allow your body to absorb the training stress and make the necessary cellular adaptations to become stronger.

You'll need to allocate time in your schedule to meet the daily training goals. This might mean waking up earlier to get your training run in before heading off to work. Also, select a day, usually Saturday or Sunday, when you can make time for a two- to four-hour-long aerobic run each week.

Plan for the weather. If you are scheduled to run a fall marathon, you'll be training in the summer. Plan your long runs and hard training sessions for the coolest times of the day. Check the weather forecast during your training and strategize your sessions. The same goes for the winter months if you're training for a spring marathon . . . dress appropriately (a few layers!) and plan your workouts for the warmest times of day.

Invest in your body. Since you've already invested in this race with the entry fee, your shoes, and your travel expenses, you should book your sports massage therapy appointments now. One massage a month should do the trick. Receiving sports massage therapy on a regular basis increases your chances of a successful, injury-free marathon buildup.

Run on trails as much as possible. The marathon will likely be on pavement, but doing most of your training runs on trails or dirt paths could help minimize the impact forces caused by running and the risk of injury during the training cycle. If you live in an area with limited access to trails, then invest in some cushy shoe insoles from your local running store.

Keep your training runs enjoyable. Mix in some different types of training runs during your marathon buildup. Venture out and explore new routes; download some new music to listen to during your workouts; tackle hills, flats, and everything in between; or simply run with new people to help beat the boredom caused by doing the same-old, same-old.

If you do your long runs alone, it might be a great idea to download an audiobook or podcast and learn a little something along the way. Just one caveat: If you run in the city or on a bike path, keep the volume low enough so that you can hear vehicular or bike traffic coming toward you.

Know that marathon training ebbs and flows. Some weeks will be great and feel easy, while others will inevitably be a struggle. Some mornings you'll wake up feeling energized, ready to tackle a long run, and other mornings you'll stay in bed a little longer than you meant to (it's so cozy!). It's all a good lesson for the race itself, though. Even when you have a challenging minute (or mile), you can trust that there will be a positive stretch ahead as well.

ASK A PRO

SARAH ATTAR, TWO-TIME OLYMPIC MARATHONER

What advice would you give to first-time marathoners?

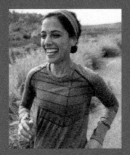

Part of the draw of running a marathon is the intimidation factor. It may be farther than you've ever run, and you know it will be difficult, but you also know that it's possible. A phrase I continually keep in mind is "respect the long run." I find myself repeating this phrase in big training blocks before Sunday's long run and before the race. It reminds me of that intimidation factor, that I am about to take on this big daunting thing, but it also has this element of confidence and understanding. When we acknowledge the grandeur, we acknowledge that this task will command the best from us, allowing us to properly prepare and approach. With this phrase in mind, I find myself staying on top of sleep, eating the right foods the night before, putting in the necessary miles to be as prepared as possible, and really paying attention to all of the details in training that will allow me to honor this race.

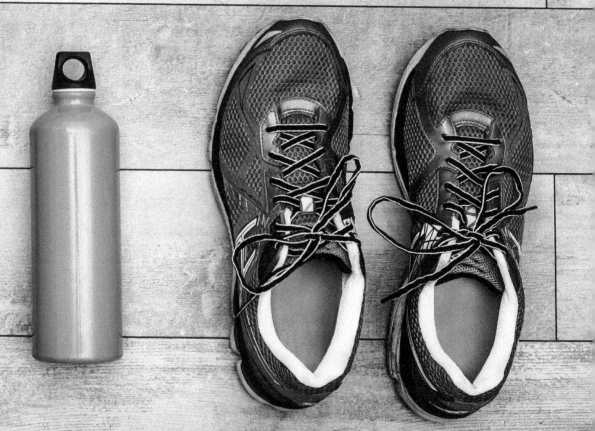

2

RUNNING GEAR

Being comfortable and well prepared during marathon training is an absolute must. And there's a reason that apparel is a giant subset of the running gear industry: Everyone is always on the hunt for the perfect solution to some issue or other. There are seamlessly constructed tights and shorts (reduces or eliminates chafing), compression socks (helps with blood flow), jackets with a durable water repellent (DWR) coating (keeps you dry without overheating in the rain), and more. The technology keeps getting better and better, and there could seriously be an entire book dedicated to running apparel, but I am going to keep it short and sweet. I get asked a lot of questions about gear when I host running clinics, so I'm highlighting advice on some of the topics that seem to come up most frequently.

The point of this book is not to sell you on any one item in particular, but rather to inform you that there are a lot of things on the market that could theoretically assist you along your marathon-training journey. You don't have to literally run out and buy any of the items I will be discussing in this chapter. In fact, one of the best facts about running is that you really don't need much gear or to spend much money, to get started at all. And just because something has a higher price tag attached to it does not automatically mean it's better or going to make you faster. My goal is to simply enlighten you on the potential benefits of some of the most popular running gear available these days.

YOUR OWN TWO FEET

Being in the business of coaching elite runners, I have seen all types of feet on some of the best marathoners in the world. Take two-time Olympic marathoner Ryan Hall, for example. His feet have extremely high arches. Then, on the opposite side of the arch-height spectrum is four-time Olympic Marathoner Meb Keflezighi, who has rather flat feet. To me, this is solid proof that the size and shape of your foot should not dictate how far or fast you can run.

In fact, each of us have feet that were uniquely created just for us. Each one contains 26 bones, held together by ligaments, fascia, retinaculum, and skin. The foot is reasonably flexible and pliable by itself, but when it's loaded with your body weight, it becomes a ridge lever to help propel your body forward, which plays an essential role in walking and running.

There is no type of foot that is best for marathon running, but there are several characteristics of a foot that can affect how you run, such as arch height, toe-spread ability, and pronation (or supination).

Arch Height

The three classifications of arch height are: high (your arches are rigid), normal (your arches aren't too rigid or too flexible), and flat (your arches are really flexible). People with flat, or low arches, typically have the most problems with overuse injuries, but that is not to say it's a given that they're going to have issues.

Pronation

You've probably heard the term *pronation* before. In short, it is the inward roll of your foot upon landing, or striking the ground. Pronation is your body's natural way of protecting your foot and softening the impact when you run and walk. However, depending on your foot type and running style, many people tend to either over-pronate (foot turns farther inward upon landing, tends to occur with runners with flatter arches) or supinate (foot turns outward upon landing, tends to be runners with higher arches).

Toe-Spread Ability

Having the ability to splay your toes out from one another is something that could help you as a runner. Some people are blessed with dexterity in their toes, meaning they can wiggle them individually, which helps keep your feet healthy and strong. Runners with this trait can recruit the small muscles that assist the movement of each toe, meaning that the intrinsic stabilizer muscles between the bones of their feet stay strong and active during long grueling training sessions and on rocky, uneven trails.

WHAT TO LOOK FOR IN A NEW PAIR OF RUNNING SHOES

As I mentioned earlier in the book, you will log about 700 miles in the process of training for your marathon. That's a lot of foot strikes, about 1,600 (800 each foot) per each one-mile run! What you wear on your feet will play an essential role in keeping you strong and injury-free throughout the season. One of the most important things you'll do before starting your training plan will be to get fitted for a comfortable, appropriate pair of running shoes. My advice is to walk into your local running store and ask a sales associate for a few recommendations for you based on your foot type, running gait (how you take off and land), and training goals. Then try each of them on, run around the store a little bit, and see what feels best. They watch people run in new shoes multiple times per day and will be able to help guide you.

Expert Mike McKeeman, manager of Bryn Mawr Running Company in Bryn Mawr, Pennsylvania, shares some pointers for next time you're on the hunt.

1. FUNCTION: The biggest challenge when choosing a running shoe is matching the function of the shoe to your individual foot type. The first step is figuring out what category of shoe you're looking for:

Stability: These are supportive shoes, designed for runners who overpronate, which tends to occur most commonly among people with flat arches and can potentially lead to many common running injuries, such as knee or shin pain, but stability shoes are designed to help correct this motion. Stability shoes will have a dense foam or plastic post on the medial side of the shoe to prevent your arch from collapsing inward. These firmer portions of the shoe keep the foot in a more neutral gait, with a normal amount of pronation.

Neutral: This category is made for runners who have strong or high arches and do not need correction for overpronation. These runners often supinate. Supination is not nearly as common as overpronation, but it can also increase injury risk in some cases. Neutral shoes feature soles that are made with foam of the same density on all sides, allowing the foot to continue using its natural and proper pronation. They are often more cushioned than stability shoes to help provide comfort to rigid, high arches, as well.

Motion Control: Shoes in this category are essentially stability shoes taken to the extreme. These stiff, rigid, incredibly stable shoes are typically reserved for runners who have supremely flat feet and overpronate to drastic levels. Made with highly dense foams and even more plastic posting than the most structured stability shoes, they help guide the most severe overpronators back to a more neutral position, working to potentially lower their risk of injury.

2. FIT: Your running shoes should fit your feet differently from your other shoes. Your foot will swell and expand throughout a long run, so there should be about a thumbnail-sized space between the front of your longest toe and the end of your shoe. Failure to have enough space in the front of your shoes can cause blisters, black toenails, and general discomfort. Your running shoes should also fit snugly around the heel and midfoot so your foot is secure and not slipping. However, it's also nice to have some extra width in the toe box (at the top of the shoe where toes sit), so your toes can splay out as your foot hits the ground. While a snug fit can be a good thing, your shoes shouldn't feel tight. Keep in mind that you most likely wear a larger size in running shoes than you do in casual shoes, typically a half or a full size bigger.

3. FORM: Many runners have heard of "barefoot running," but the concept is often misunderstood. Studies have shown that the most efficient way to run is the way we run when we are barefoot: landing on our midfoot, with our toes splayed out. It is our most natural state of movement. Without shoes on, our forefoot and heel are level on the ground—not stacked, as they often are in running shoes. Our natural gait should have us landing close to that same position.

Traditionally, most running shoes have featured an elevated heel to give more cushioning to the heel than the forefoot, so there is a drop in height from heel to forefoot. In the shoe industry, that height difference is referred to as heel-to-toe drop. On stability shoes, the heel-to-toe drop is about 12 mm. However, most shoe companies have recently begun lowering the drop on their shoes to promote a more efficient, barefoot-like running gait. These shoes still contain plenty of cushioning, but put your foot in a better position when landing. Many shoes now feature a drop in the 8- to 10-mm range, while others go as low as 4 to 6 mm. Some companies are even producing

shoes with a 0-mm drop, meaning the shoe is exactly level from heel to forefoot. Being aware of the heel-to-toe drop of your shoes could help you find the level that is best for your foot and running style.

4. FEEL: Running shoes can feel soft, firm, or something in between. Some people love to feel like they're running on marshmallows, while others prefer to feel the ground underneath them a bit more. Keep in mind that a firm shoe can give you just as much cushioning and shock absorption as a soft shoe, just with a different feeling underfoot. There are varying degrees of cushioning—maximum, mid-level, and low—within each category of shoe (except for flats, which are all minimal). The amount of cushioning provided will directly affect the amount of shock absorption you're getting from the shoe. One thing to consider is that if you've had Achilles problems in the past, then you will probably be better off with a firmer shoe. When you wear a soft shoe, your heel sinks further into the foam, which can put more strain on your heel and foot.

5. FASHION: For some people, this may be the number-one priority, but in reality, it should be the last thing to consider when choosing a shoe. When you have more than one shoe that seems to work well for your foot in terms of function, fit, form, and feel, however, you can absolutely use fashion as your tiebreaker. After all, we all know that if you look good, you'll feel good, and if you feel good, you may have a more enjoyable run. Just make sure you don't allow fashion to dictate your feelings about everything else.

WHEN TO UPDATE YOUR SHOES

Just like all good things, your running shoes must also come to an end, and once a pair is past its prime, your risk of injury and discomfort increases. You need to swap your shoes out regularly because the midsole inevitably breaks down, causing the shoes to lose their structure and not protect your feet against the impact of running.

So when is the right time to replace your favorite pair? First, the obvious: Look at the wear and tear on its rubber tread, or outsole. Second, running shoes typically have a lifespan of about 300 to 500 miles, depending on a runner's bio-mechanical efficiency (if you strike the ground harder or overpronate/supinate more often, you're going to beat up your shoes more quickly).

DRESS FOR SUCCESS

When coaches say "dress for success," it doesn't mean the same thing as when a business professor says it. Our more casual version is all about making yourself as comfortable, light, and dry as possible to improve your performance and overall enjoyment every time you go out for a run. When you start introducing long runs into your repertoire, this becomes even more important, since you'll be spending even more time wearing that gear out on the road.

Socks

Running socks play a key role in how your feet transfer their power to the road. Most importantly, they need to work with the shoes you're wearing to maximize comfort and performance. A sock's main purpose is to help prevent excessive rubbing of your foot against your shoe and prevent blisters. If blisters do form, they can lead to poor mechanics while you run and cause a lot of discomfort. When selecting running socks, try a few different pairs to see what feels best with the shoes you're currently running in. You can opt for ergonomically correct L- and R-footed socks—which feel great but can complicate your laundry—or go simple. To me, the simpler, the better. Thin, breathable socks that feature extra cushioning on the heel and forefoot and fit snugly against my feet seem to work well and complement most running shoe styles.

Sports Bras

These should clearly be supportive, breathable, and comfortable. In general, look for one that is designed specifically for high-impact activities (no yoga bras!) and is a good fit for you personally. Once again, the staff at your local running store could be a tremendous help in this department, and reading online reviews before buying a bra is always advised.

ESSENTIAL ACCESSORIES

Sometimes it's the little things that make the biggest difference when out on a run. Investing in the right accessories could help keep you warm, cool, dry, connected, and most importantly, safe, out on the road.

Bracing for the Cold

In the winter, some of the most useful accessories will be face masks, gloves, high cotton socks, running pants, and water-resistant jackets. Your main goals in layering up during this season are to protect your skin, stay warm and dry, and keep your digits from going numb. I have also become accustomed to smearing a thin layer of petroleum jelly or Vaseline on my face to keep it moist and add a thin layer of protection from the dry, cold winter air.

If you live somewhere with snow or ice in the winter, then you'll also need extra traction on your shoes. One accessory that I use all the time here in the Sierra Mountains is Yaktrax, which are basically removable cables with chains for your running shoes. They are easy to install (much, much easier than installing actual car tire chains or cables), and you can put them right on your regular running shoes in a matter of seconds. One of the best things about these is that if you start your run off in icy or snowy conditions, and then come to a dry stretch of road, you can simply remove the cables and reinstall them later if needed.

Running in the Dark

If you tend to do evening or early-morning runs, then it's a good idea to invest in a headlamp for running in the dark. Otherwise, roots, rocks, and curbs are lurking at every mile and could trip you up if you're not prepared. A small, lightweight headlamp usually costs $15 to $30, and its batteries can be easily changed out every few weeks, or you can purchase a slightly more expensive (but way more convenient) rechargeable one.

Reflectors are a must-have when training in the dark. Make sure you have one on your back and front. Running clothes often have pops of reflectivity on them as well, which can be a good way to help make yourself more visible to drivers who might be slightly checked out, sipping on their morning lattes on their way to work.

Staying Hydrated

Staying hydrated is essential when you're out on long runs, so bring your own H_2O along for the ride. You'll want to have a good water bottle or hydration pack to sip from throughout your training. And remember, it should be filled with the same kind of fluid that's going to be served during the race you're training for.

When looking for a hydration pack, keep in mind that smaller and lighter is often better. You won't want anything that will weigh you down while you run. There's a wide range of fluid volume sizes available. A two-liter (70 oz.) pack will be plenty for a three- to four-hour run. Handheld water bottles are helpful, too. Carrying a bottle of water can seem a bit cumbersome after a few miles, so you might want to consider stashing it in the bushes and then circling back when you need a drink, giving your arms a tiny break.

Listening to Music

Back in the 1990s, I used to run with a Sony Walkman, listening to a mixtape that I recorded off an FM station (KROQ) in Southern California. Ha! My, how times have changed. Audio devices have gotten much smaller and lighter, with an enormous memory capacity, so you can basically have every song in your personal library at your fingertips while you work out. Running while listening to music is obviously a personal preference, but it can be an etiquette issue as well.

Training with a group of runners while listening to music is a social faux pas. Listening to music while running alone on the treadmill, however, is just fine. Some race organizations, such as the New York Road Runners (NYRR), frown upon the use of personal headphones for safety reasons. Here's a snippet from NYRR's Rules of Competition page in their Help Center: "The use of headphones is strongly discouraged. If you must wear headphones, be extra-aware of your surroundings and make sure you can hear announcements as well as being aware of other participants around you."

Research shows that listening to music while training could have a performance-enhancing effect. I know this was true when my wife, Deena, was undergoing physiological performance testing at the Olympic Training Center in Chula Vista, California. Michael Shannon, head exercise physiologist at the center, would blast Deena's favorite techno beats through a surround-sound stereo system to get her to give her absolute maximum effort on the treadmill during the testing protocol, and it worked.

Protecting Your Eyes

Sunglasses are an essential part of my running attire, and I've been wearing them on my runs for the last 25 years. I wear sunglasses every single day for a couple of reasons. First, they help protect my eyes from small bugs, dust, and other particles in the air that the wind might kick up. Second, they're a performance enhancer. When I was in high school, a coach once told me that sunglasses reduce upper body tension when running. He went into the mechanics of why: When we squint our eyes due to the brightness of the sun, that tension sets off a chain reaction beginning with the recruitment and contraction of the muscles in our face. The "tensing up" effect trickles down to the muscles in our necks and ultimately leads to the shoulder muscles becoming contracted, which thus restricts their range of motion. And as the song goes, "Heads, shoulders, knees, and toes." In other words, tension up top has a direct influence on everything below as well.

GADGETS

Gadgets now play a role in all sports, especially in running. We have watches that tell us how long, fast, and far we've run. We have wireless heart-rate monitors, too. This information can then be downloaded to a device so you can analyze your stats whenever you want. With some smart watches, runners can even answer their phones mid-run if need be.

The following are some go-to gadgets for runners.

A chronograph stopwatch with 50-lap counter is about the simplest way to go in terms of choosing a watch. I have been using a Timex running watch off and on for 25 years. This easy-to-use wrist piece tells me the amount of time I've been running and can record each lap split time from a track workout, too. I have run four marathons with this type of watch, gauging my pace off each mile marker on the course for real-time feedback.

Watches that use a global positioning system (GPS) provide instant feedback regarding your pace, while at the same time displaying how far into your run you currently are. Many GPS watches can sync up with your computer or your phone to graph the elevation and map every course you've run, too.

Recovery gadgets, such as foam rollers or stick-type devices, are no substitute for massage therapy, but they sure come close. These DIY rollers can help push lactic acid out post-workout, break up your myofascia (tissue between your muscles), and help speed up the entire recovery process. For decades, athletes have been rolling out their own muscle kinks and knots to reduce muscle tightness. A few notable recovery devices out there are the ROLL Recovery R8, which uses a gentle clamp-type device to press rollerblade wheels against large muscle groups; foam rollers, which you press against your tissue, using your own body weight; and the Stick, which pretty much describes itself.

The almighty treadmill is the ultimate gadget to assist in your training! Or, as some runners affectionately refer to it, "the dreadmill." Treadmills can come in handy when the weather outside is frightful, either snowy or scorching hot. Low-end treadmills cost $300 to $500, while top-end versions can seriously be comparable in price to a compact car, nearing the $20,000 price tag. More expensive treadmills are usually better products. In addition to giving you an indoor option for your training runs, treadmills also help cushion the impact forces of running and can help facilitate either a nice, flat recovery run or a hilly one, simply by adjusting the incline.

POPULAR APPS FOR RUNNERS

If you like to track every step of your training while listening to music, chart your weight loss, or "compete" against other runners, you might want to consider downloading one of these popular running apps to your smartphone. You'll need to carry your phone with you when you're training for most of these apps to work.

Runner's World Go: Provides expert knowledge and motivation you need to "absolutely crush it."

Strava: Serves as a complete tracking service via GPS that you can share with your friends or the running community in general. Other runners on this platform will be able to view your routes and compete against your times.

MapMyRun: One of the first running apps ever created, this app provides useful information for running in new cities or finding new routes in your own town.

ASK A PRO

JANE HUBBARD, 6:00 MARATHONER

What's the one piece of gear you would recommend to a first-time marathoner?

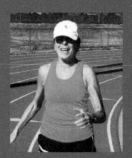

I *need* my watch! My watch is very basic. It tells time, keeps continuous time from race start to finish, and times each mile. Pace is the most important thing. You have to pace yourself properly to be able to finish 26.2 miles without hitting the wall. Your mind is going to get tired as time passes. Don't make your timing complicated! All you have to do is remember to press the lap button, and your watch will display your time for the previous mile. This keeps you from starting out too fast and gives you a little nudge as you tire toward the end of the race. Based on your training runs and advice from your coach, decide on a realistic pace. Then adjust your effort based on the mile you just ran. Keep it simple. You will thank me later.

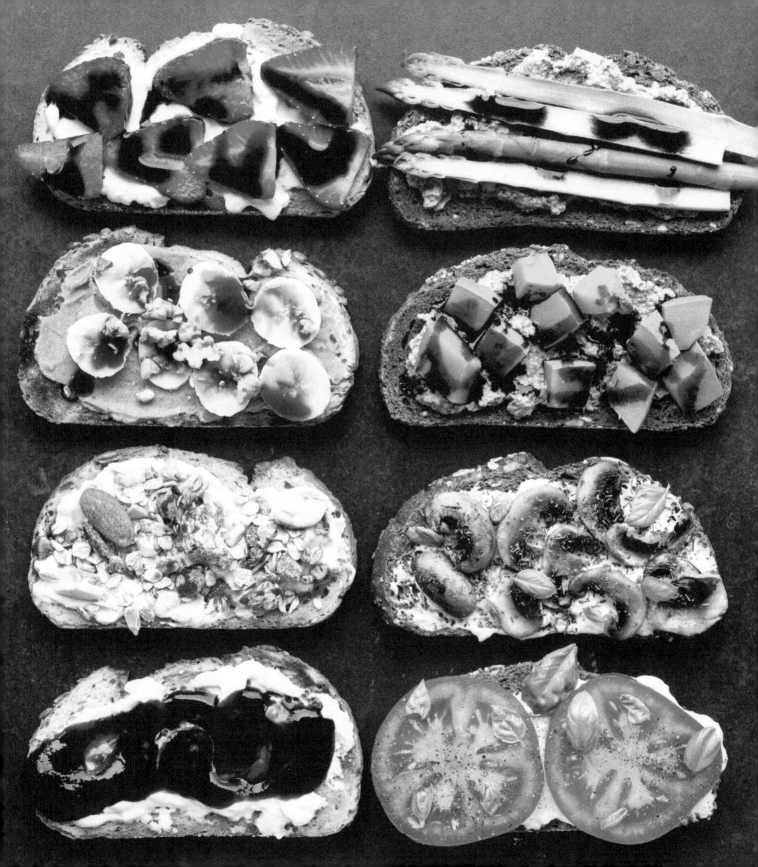

3

FUELING YOUR BODY

When I was in college, training, competing, and studying, I paid little attention to what I needed to consume between workouts to help with my recovery. Let's face it, my diet was pretty poor, consisting of way too many bowls of cereal per day and a large plate of spaghetti for dinner. Where were the fruits and vegetables? Where was the lean protein? I honestly don't know how I ever made it through in one piece.

The adage "You are what you eat" really holds true. If you want to do extraordinary things, you can't eat ordinary food! Marathon runners need to eat exceptionally well, consuming a variety of vegetables, fruits, and lean meats, to perform at their best and help reduce their risk of injury. You can't expect to have a high-quality run or race if you're putting low-quality (or not enough) food in your body.

This chapter will cover nutrition, serving to both inform and guide you on the different types of food choices you should make as a runner. Making smart decisions to stay nourished during periods of heavy training is critical to your end results. Something as basic as opting for a midday snack, like fruit, which is rich in vitamins and electrolytes, over a nutrient-poor Snickers bar, for example, will add up over time and cause noticeable changes in your body and training. One common mistake is to confuse thirst for hunger, so carrying a refillable water bottle around with you everywhere and sipping throughout the day will help you stay hydrated and satiated.

TYPES OF FUEL

In the beginning of your marathon training, you will notice a spike in your metabolism (increased calorie burn) after just a couple of weeks of running. Your caloric needs will be more demanding than normal, and probably higher than those around you who are not running several miles a day, so you'll need to eat more food, more frequently. Your body will be burning lots of calories during your training sessions, but it will also be burning calories afterward, during the so-called "after-burn," or a few hours post-workout. A runner's physique has the tendency to refine itself to the most efficient shape over the course of a training cycle, but only when that athlete is using high-quality fuel.

The United States Department of Agriculture (USDA) has been evolving their Food Wheels, Food Pyramids, Basic Four Daily Food Guides, Hassle-Free Food Guides, and MyPlate graphics since the 1940s, to educate our society on how much of each food group to eat each day. But I'm here to tell you that it doesn't need to be super complicated. In fact, following a marathoner's diet is simple: You'll need plenty of carbohydrates, fat, and protein to fuel your workouts, but these can come in all sorts of delicious forms. The main sources will be whole foods, consisting of vegetables, proteins, fruits, grains, and dairy (my wife would of course add wine to this list as well).

Below is a list of the nutrients that marathon runners need to meet their energy demands for achieving peak performance on a daily basis. These nutrients are needed to both supply energy and for recovery.

CARBOHYDRATES (grains, pasta, potatoes)

*Shoot for 60–65% of your total caloric intake.

Training 60–120 minutes/day: 3–4.5 grams of carbohydrates/pound or 6-9 grams/kilogram of body weight.

PROTEINS (eggs, meats)

*Aim for 15–20% of your total caloric intake.

Range: 0.5 to 0.7 grams of protein/pound or 1.2 to 2.0 grams/kilogram of body weight.

FATS (oils)

*Try to minimize at 15–25% of your total caloric intake.

Approximately 0.5 grams of fat/pound or 1 to 1.5 gram/kilogram of body weight.

Take the numbers you came up with based on your body weight and plug them into the formula below.

(Grams of carbohydrates x 4 calories/gram)
+ (Grams of protein x 4 calories/gram)
+ (Grams of fat ["the good kind"] x 9 calories/gram)

= The estimated total calories/day that are needed for sustaining your endurance activities.

Vegetables

Eat a variety of veggies—the darker the green or orange, the better, in terms of nutrient density. Veggies can be eaten raw or cooked, but the uncooked ones are going to contain more nutrients, since cooking breaks some of them down and they evaporate when heated. The common recommendation is to eat five servings of fruits and vegetables every day, which will not only positively impact your training and recovery, but also prolong your life (no big deal).

So why are vegetables so great for us runners? Well, they help us meet the high-caloric demands of training and assist in the process of building and repairing muscle, tendons, and bones and replenishing hormones that are depleted during heavy training periods.

Proteins

Runners are constantly breaking down muscle tissue during training, and a continuous intake of protein is required to help repair it all, since protein is the building block of the body, and its main function is to rebuild and restore all of our tissues (skin, bone, muscle, etc.). Proteins are made up of amino acids, and your body needs 22 different amino acids to function, 13 of which we can only naturally manufacture. So the other nine need to be consumed in the form of various foods, such as beans, grains, meats, dairy, and nuts, each day. Lean proteins, such as beans, eggs, fish, and chicken (or other white meats), should therefore be an essential part of your diet.

If you don't eat meat, that's okay. Many runners are vegetarians, pescatarians, or vegans. You will just have to work diligently to make sure you're getting enough protein in your diet, in whatever forms are possible. Ultra-runner extraordinaire Scott Jurek runs 100-plus miles a week and takes home titles from some of the most prestigious ultra-endurance races around the globe all while successfully maintaining a vegan lifestyle. His book, *Eat & Run*, goes into more detail about how he manages to maintain this balance.

Dairy

Dairy products are not only another delicious source of protein, but they also provide a great source of calcium, which plays a pivotal role in bone maintenance and development. Calcium is a mineral that plays a unique role in muscle contraction and relaxation during training. I'm personally not a fan of milk (why are we the only mammals still consuming it past our infancy?), but, I love cheese.

Fruit

Fruit contains natural sugars or carbohydrates and is another key ingredient to a successful marathon-training season. Along with giving our bodies energy, they provide nutrients that assist in maintaining an active lifestyle. All fruits contain electrolytes, which help with muscle contractions. Here's a list of some of my favorite fruits that are packed with electrolytes: bananas, oranges, kiwi, avocado, tomatoes, and nectarines.

Grains

Grains, or what were once referred to as the "breads, rice, and pasta group" on the Food Guide Pyramid, are derived from oats, wheat, barley, or cornmeal. These whole foods are high in complex carbohydrates, which are incredibly useful for endurance activities and can help with the complete digestive process, thanks to their added fiber. These are far different from the nutrient-poor, simple sugars found in cookies and candy.

Sugars

One thing you should steer clear of as a runner is refined sugar. Simple sugars, in the form of refined sugars, are just empty calories (in that they provide no nutritional value) that your body uses for energy. They are absent of vitamins, minerals, antioxidants, proteins. and fats. Frequent spikes in sugar consumption can throw off our blood sugar regulatory hormone, insulin. The irregular production of this hormone can cause problems when you run for a long distance, as your body is trying to use both carbohydrates and fats as fuel for sustained and lasting energy, and it can become a bit confused as to which substrate to use for energy production.

HOW TO EAT LIKE A RUNNER

Over the course of my running career, I have experimented with different types of prerace and pre-workout meals, and what I've learned is that the perfect meal seems to evolve throughout my life. What worked for me in high school is not necessarily what works for me today. The reason I'm telling you this is so you understand that there's not one solution or meal for the masses. Keep in mind that it will take time to figure out what meals work best for you during training.

Here are a few things to keep in mind when planning your meal:

1. Your pre-run meal should be consumed one to two hours before you start your training run.

2. A small, post-run recovery meal should be consumed 30 to 60 minutes after the workout.

3. Eat frequent, small meals (five to seven) throughout the day to keep your blood sugar level up.

4. Make a general outline of what you are going to eat during the day so that you strategically plan to get a variety foods in.

5. Rather than simply increasing your caloric intake to match energy demands, you should focus on increasing the nutrient quality of your diet. This means there needs to be a decrease in the consumption of low-quality foods, like white bread, candy, and packaged products.

But how do you know how much to eat? Don't worry, you do not need to get a little food scale to

Caffeine and Alcohol

I love my coffee, but too much caffeine and marathon training do not necessarily mix. While caffeinated coffee is considered a performance-enhancing supplement, since it gives your central nervous system a boost and power to mobilize free fatty acids, it also has a dehydrating effect. So whenever I ramp up my training for a half-marathon or marathon, I concentrate on eliminating my afternoon cup of coffee and reducing my morning intake to just one 8-ounce cup. I also replace that afternoon cup of coffee with a very large bottle of water, which helps keep me hydrated.

Alcohol is another one of my vices, but again, everything is best in moderation, especially when training. My wife and I love to open a bottle of wine in the evenings and have a glass (or two) while we prepare our dinner, but too much of anything can be detrimental to meeting your training goals. Red wine has health benefits, since it contains vitamins and anti-oxidants, which make having one glass an evening justifiable, even during peak marathon training! In August 2004, my wife ran the Women's Olympic Marathon in Athens, Greece, after having a glass of wine with dinner the night before, and she took home the bronze medal. Perhaps it would have been even shinier, if not for the wine? Or maybe the wine enhanced her performance by having a soothing, relaxing effect? Truth is, we'll never know.

And it's not just wine. Beer and cocktails can be okay, too, so long as they are consumed in small amounts and relative to your tolerance. But remember, the effects of alcohol on athletic performance are usually negative. Drinking excessive alcohol (four to five drinks) in one evening can have a detrimental effect on your running performance for up to three days.

weigh each meal, as former (defrocked) cycling champion Lance Armstrong notoriously used to do. I believe that eating slowly and chewing your food well will automatically and instinctively control your portion sizes.

Your pre-workout meal should contain 200 to 400 calories and be comprised of 60 to 70% carbohydrates and 30 to 40% split between fats and protein. If you eat two hours beforehand, you can eat more, closer to 300 to 400 calories. However, if you're only eating one hour beforehand, then scale that back down to around 200 calories (one slice of whole wheat toast, a tablespoon of peanut butter, and half of a banana, sliced).

As for your post-workout meal, you'll want to consume a combination of protein and carbohydrates to help repair broken-down tissues and replenish your glycogen stores (carbs that are stored in muscle tissue). It pays to plan ahead with your recovery meals. The timing of this meal is just as important as the pre-workout one. Eating within 30 to 60 minutes after you finish your workout is the best way to absorb the calories. This meal doesn't need to fill you up—it simply needs to satiate your appetite until you eat another meal just a couple of hours later.

Keep in mind that when running, you'll burn an average of 100 to 120 calories per mile, regardless of pace. The biggest factor in determining calories burned per mile is the size of the runner, not his or her pace. Men typically burn more calories during exercise, due to their greater lean muscle mass and the fact that they generally weigh more than women. Another factor to consider is age—the older the athlete, the fewer calories they will burn. RunnersConnect has a calculator to judge how many calories you'll need to burn at www.runnersconnect.net/training/tools/calorie-calculator.

Nobody likes to be hangry (or to be around someone else who is), so I advise you to carry an easy and delicious snack with you at all times when you're marathon training. You never know when you might get a sudden hankering for a PB&J with banana slices. It's better to be prepared than barred by your loved ones from ever training for a marathon again.

FIVE RUNNER-FRIENDLY FOODS

1. WHOLE-GRAIN PASTA can be a great source of complex carbohydrates, the type of fuel all marathon runners need. There's a reason that race organizations traditionally host a "Pasta Dinner" the night before their race, as this meal provides much-needed energy just hours before the gun goes off. Pasta is easily digestible and can be garnished with a light marinara or butter sauce. Pairing it with some sort of lean protein is often recommended for a healthy prerace meal. You should practice your prerace meal in training, eating the exact same thing the night before a few of your long runs, so that you know how your body responds to everything before you reach the starting line.

2. BLUEBERRIES are a known superfood, full of disease-fighting antioxidants, vitamins, minerals, and fiber. They also help fight inflammation and can speed up post-workout recovery. With these qualities, it's no wonder they now seem to be on runners' radars.

3. BANANAS are my personal favorite fruit. My pre-workout breakfast always incorporates a banana or two. They are easily digestible, providing a regulatory effect on your digestive tract. Plus, they provide energy in the form of carbohydrates and loads of potassium to help assist with muscle contraction.

4. STEAK, or another type of red meat, can help keep your iron levels up. I know, I know, it is not a lean meat, but consuming red meat just once or twice a week is a good way to up your iron. Repeated foot-strike impact on the ground during running has been found to lower iron levels in our blood through a process called *hemolysis*. Runners need to be conscious of this phenomenon and combat it with consumption of iron-rich foods, such as steak.

5. PEANUT BUTTER is another fantastic food for runners in training. Not only is it delicious, but peanut butter also contains protein and the best antioxidant readily available to us, vitamin E. This powerful antioxidant fights against damaging oxidative agents (free radicals) that the body produces naturally.

FIVE PERFORMANCE-ENHANCING SNACKS

1. PEANUT BUTTER AND JELLY SANDWICH WITH BANANA SLICES: Not only does this bring back fond childhood memories, but it also provides a good amount of carbohydrates, protein, and fiber.

2. TUNA FISH SANDWICH ON WHOLE-WHEAT BREAD: This classic is a wonderful mashup of exceptional sources of protein and fiber.

3. FRUIT SMOOTHIE: Made with yogurt, berries, and juice, this drink is an excellent source of protein, carbohydrates, calcium, antioxidants, and vitamins, and is great when you're on the go.

4. RAW VEGGIES DIPPED IN LOW-FAT DRESSING: This is quick and healthy snack that's super convenient when you have less than one minute in your day to prepare something nutritious to eat!

5. CUP OF CHICKEN NOODLE SOUP AND CRACKERS: This warm snack is a great source of protein, carbohydrates, and sodium—perfect for cold winter days.

ASK A PRO

MONICA PRELLE, MEMBER OF THE MAMMOTH TRACK CLUB WITH A 2:56 MARATHON PERSONAL RECORD

What's your favorite recipe or snack for runners?

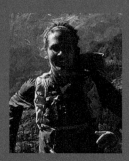

Marathon training inevitably makes me tired and hungry—all the time—so I like to keep the house stocked with a lot of healthy foods that are quick and easy to prepare. When I get home from a run and I need to eat something immediately, I make a recovery smoothie that includes natural anti-inflammatory ingredients: cucumber, ginger, pineapple, and water with Vega Sport vanilla protein powder or plain Greek yogurt. My go-to snack plate between meals includes fresh-milk mozzarella, prosciutto, and seasonal fresh fruit like a Pink Lady apple or white peaches. For lunches I make good use of dinner leftovers. My favorite is quinoa and steak tossed with cucumber, red onion, avocado, red pepper, and extra-virgin olive oil (served cold). For general snacking, I always have roasted pistachios on hand. I'm also a big fan of GoMacro Cashew Carmel bars and take them everywhere with me in case of a hunger emergency.

STAY HYDRATED!

Our bodies are made up of 60 to 70% water, so it's no wonder that it's such an important part of our existence. While we can go a week or two without food, we certainly can't go without water for more than a few days. It's needed for every single cellular process; moistening the mouth, nose, and eyes; lubricating our joints; keeping the digestive system regular; and helping to filter out waste by-products from respiration.

Being hydrated is key when starting a training run. But sometimes it can be hard to know if you're properly hydrated. Before you start your run, use the restroom and check the color of your urine. If it's almost clear, then you are sufficiently hydrated and may proceed with your training run. However, if it has a yellow tint or you haven't had to use the bathroom since waking in the morning, then it would be wise to wait until you've consumed 8 to 10 ounces of water before you make your way out the door.

During training, consuming water cools your body in the same way that radiator coolant regulates the temperature of a car's engine. It's essential to refill your bodily fluid levels hourly by sipping water throughout the day. For every 1% drop in body weight from fluid loss, there is a 2% drop in running performance. The loss of 3.5 pounds in a runner weighing 120 pounds means a 6% decrease in performance, which adds up to several minutes over the course of a marathon.

The American Council on Exercise has suggested the following basic guidelines for drinking water before, during, and after exercise:

Drink 17 to 20 ounces of water, two to three hours before you start exercising.

Drink 8 ounces of water 20 to 30 minutes before you start exercising or during your warmup.

Drink 7 to 10 ounces of water every 10 to 20 minutes during exercise.

Drink 8 ounces of water no more than 30 minutes after you finish exercising.

To figure out how much water you're losing through sweat, and therefore, how much you should be replacing as a result, use this formula from Cathy Utzschneider's *Mastering Running*:

1. Weigh yourself nude before a run.

2. Run (at race pace) for one hour. Do not drink during that hour.

3. After the run, reweigh yourself nude, having toweled off sweat.

4. Subtract your weight after the run from your weight before the run and convert to ounces.

5. To determine how much you should drink about every 15 minutes, divide that number by four. If you have lost 32 ounces, drink about 8 ounces of fluid every 15 minutes.

6. Because the test reflects sweat loss based on environmental conditions that day, repeat the test under different conditions to see how they affect your sweat rate. You'll likely get different results under different temperatures, altitudes, and paces.

Sports Drinks

So when do you need to sip on a sports drink? First, let's define the term *sports drink* as a beverage that's consumed while exercising, or pre- or post- exercise, and typically contains both electrolytes, like sodium and potassium, and carbohydrates. Sports drinks were created for the sole purpose of replenishing depleted fluids and calories that are lost through muscle contractions and sweat. They should be consumed sparingly when *not* running or exercising, since our bodies don't need the excess sugar when sedentary.

I highly recommend using a sports drink during your training runs that are over one hour in duration. A good rule of thumb is to drink about 4 to 6 ounces every 15 to 20 minutes only during your long marathon-training runs each week. Remember to research the beverage that will be served at the aid stations on your race course, and start practicing your training runs with that as soon as possible.

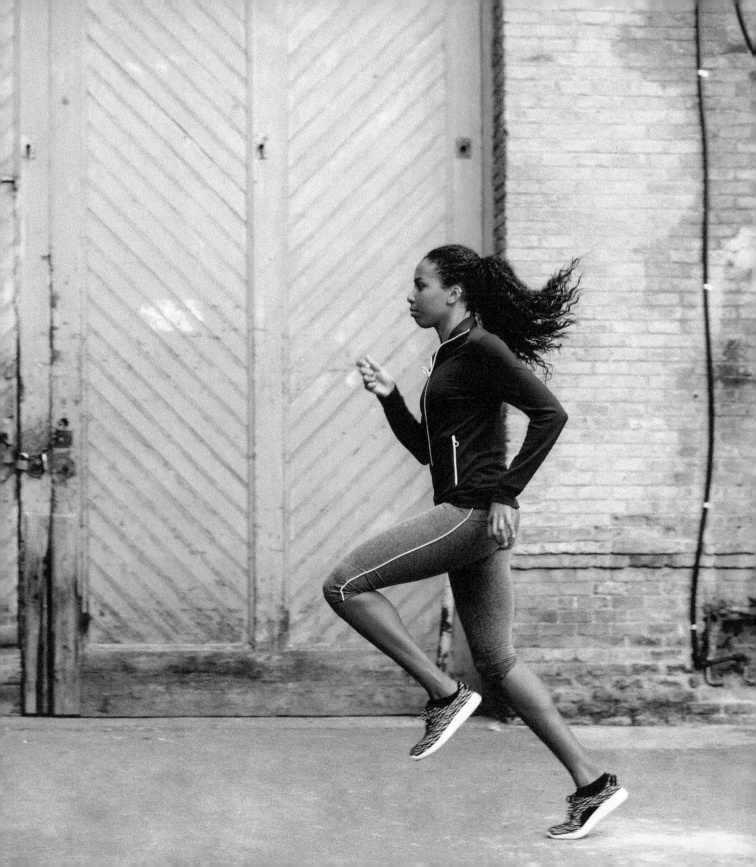

4

PROPER RUNNING FORM

Running with proper technique and form helps improve your efficiency and greatly reduces your risk of injury. Practicing good running form from day one is vital to the success of your training—and the rest of your running career, really. Some athletes are naturally blessed with having the "perfect" running form, but most of us need to put in a little work to get it just right. Always keep in mind that the human body was built for endurance and is designed to run efficiently for long distances. The code to marathon training is hidden deep inside your DNA, and all it takes is some time and effort to unlock it.

BREATHING

If you're ever out on the track in Mammoth Lakes, California, on a Tuesday morning in the summer, you are sure to hear me boisterously yelling *"Big lungs!"* to our athletes as they perform their speed work. This simple phrase is one way to encourage folks who want to improve their race performances.

Athletes who work on expanding their lungs while they run can further develop their respiratory muscles to forcefully and maximally contract, ensuring that they get every milliliter of air possible down deep into the healthy pink tissues of the lungs. That's why when an athlete asks me how they can run faster uphill, rather than saying, "Just move your legs faster and try harder," I'll say, "Breathe deeper while fostering the intention of running fast." It helps, I promise.

The Mechanics of Breathing

We have a lot of different muscles that help us breathe. While our lungs are the main component of the respiratory system and play the biggest role, they also need the surrounding muscles to help them move, to control their expansion and contraction. Some of these muscles, such as the diaphragm, which works to depress the lungs and create space that produces negative pressure and allows air to flow in to each lobe, may sound familiar. However, others like the intercostal muscles, which increase or decrease the space between your ribs to control the expansion and constriction of your rib cage, are probably less known.

We want to maximize the volume, or space, in our lungs when we run. Breathing deeply, rather than taking quick, shallow breaths, will help facilitate this goal. With shallow, rapid breathing, you lose valuable air within the respiratory system, mainly in the trachea or windpipe. Over the course of the years, I have heard lots of thoughts from other runners about what the "proper" way to breathe while running is—"Inhale for three steps, exhale for two," or "Breathe 80% through your mouth and 20% through your nose." Frankly, I've never done either of these things, and I don't think any of the athletes I coach have, either. But I believe coaches just want you to think about taking slower, deeper breaths while you stride. In my opinion, simply staying focused on breathing with "big lungs" does wonders to help maximize the workload of your biggest running engine.

During a yoga class, instructors usually place an emphasis on learning and controlling the rhythm of your breaths. They teach that the best way to breathe is with your stomach, moving your belly in and out, versus expanding with your chest. While doing yoga, a person's heart rate is typically lower than when they're running, but there is reason to consider using this breathing technique for running as well. Concentrating on using your belly for breathing will reduce the amount of stress and fatigue placed on your upper body when out for a training run. Given that we always want to keep our shoulders down and relaxed, this is one relatively easy way to stay consistent with that philosophy.

Whatever you do, do not overcomplicate your breathing technique while you're running. So long as you're expanding your lungs with every inhale and pushing out as much air as possible with every exhale, you're going to be just fine.

STRIDE

Along with keeping your breathing relaxed, having a solid stride is another way to boost your performance. Whether you're a beginner or a pro, your personal running stride is something that can continually be improved. Deena, a three-time Olympian and seasoned master's athlete, is still hearing form cues, like "Run tall" or "Keep your elbows close to your torso" from me on the sidelines. These little verbal reminders can make a difference in her stride that leads to finishing each lap a half-second faster, or slower, than usual.

When you run, you should think about doing it with your whole body. It's not just your legs moving out there. Many coaches tend to analyze how someone runs through several different phases of their natural gait: initial contact with the ground, mid-stance, take-off, initial swing, mid-swing, and terminal swing of the legs. They also pay attention to what the runner's arms are doing.

Contact and Take-Off Phases

I believe the two most important phases for you to concentrate on are the contact phase, or when your foot strikes the ground, and the take-off phase, or when you lift your knee and extend the opposing hip. During the contact phase, you should focus on striking with your midfoot rather than your heel.

And try not to bounce. Bouncing only does damage to your quad muscles and leg joints, so try to smooth out your vertical oscillation. Ideally, you should be able to balance a plate on your head while you're running.

During take-off, remember that hip extension is hugely important in propelling you forward while you run. I always like to envision a donkey standing up on his front legs and kicking out behind him with his rear legs. I will provide you with a great hip extension exercise in the next chapter, too.

Arms

What your arms do while you run is almost as important as what your legs are doing. They should be moving in concert with each other, simultaneously pumping in the opposite directions. You want to try and achieve a synchronized action between your shoulders and hips. When you pump your arms back and forth, your legs are driven forward through cleverly designed muscle and fascial tension in your abdomen. Your arms should swing freely and relaxed from your shoulders, just like a pendulum.

Head and Neck

You also want to pay close attention to what your head and neck are doing while you run. Practicing good posture (with a tall back, neutral spine, and shoulders down) is very important for both your health and performance. Running tall reduces the strain you're putting on the muscles supporting your head and spine, thus cutting down on the amount of tension you're experiencing and unnecessary energy you're expending. Your head and neck should be positioned directly over, or aligned with, your shoulders and not protracted forward, as if you were straining to see the smallest font size on your computer screen.

Tips for a Perfect Stride

Here are a few important things to look for:

Your head should be directly over your shoulders. If your head is sticking out, or you're leaning forward, your center of gravity changes, causing unnecessary tension in your Achilles tendons and the bottoms of your feet, or plantar fascia, as a result. Try standing upright, and then slowly move your head forward. Your feet and calves tighten up as you do so.

Your shoulders should be relaxed and low. Imagine dropping your shoulders down, away from your ears. If you're carrying tension in your shoulders, it limits mobility in your hips, reducing your stride efficiency.

Your elbows should be bent about 90 degrees. Remember, your arms and legs need to move at the same cadence when you run, so if the angle, or length of your arm lever, changes, so does your stride length. If the angle's smaller, your stride will be shortened; if it's larger, your stride will be extended. Either way, it will result in an inefficient gait.

Your hands should be relaxed, but not floppy. Your wrists should be rigid, meaning they don't flex or bend while you're running, and your fingers should be relaxed. As I've told thousands of runners before, just imagine

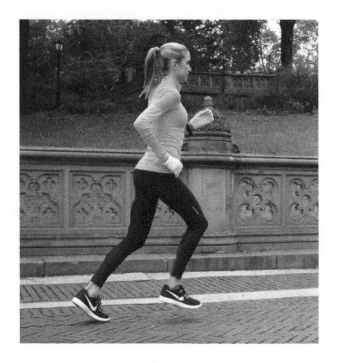

you're holding a delicate potato chip in your hand. This will keep you from clenching your fists and unnecessarily expending valuable energy.

Let your legs do their thing. Actually, don't worry too much about what anything from your hips down is doing. Just stay focused on your head and arms—the rest will fall in line with what's happening up top.

As a runner, you need to be aware of what your body is doing while you log miles (or minutes). Ask a friend, coach, or running buddy to take a short video of you running at an easy pace (ideally the pace you're aiming at for your race). This could be very helpful in determining specific ways to improve your current form.

PACE

Every record (world and American) set in the marathon in the past 20 years has been accomplished by running even, or negative, splits. What does this mean? Well, even splits occur when a runner completes the first half of the race and the second half of the race (splits) at almost the exact same pace. In other words, athletes set a goal race pace for themselves, and then maintain that steady pace throughout the course of their race. A negative split, however, occurs when runners finish the second half of the race at a pace that's faster than the first half. We can all learn from both pacing strategies and use them in our training.

Don't be deceived by the word *negative*. Negative splits generally lead to very positive results. During the 2006 London Marathon, for example, my wife's goal was to run under 2:20 for the marathon, which meant that her 5K split times needed to be right at 16:30. She started off strong, but felt good and pushed a little harder than goal race pace toward the end, giving her a negative split. However, her 5K split times deviated by less than 10 seconds each. In other words, she ran almost perfectly even, mile after mile, 5K after 5K, until she crossed the finish line.

It's very common for marathon runners to go out at a faster pace than they intended—they're motivated by the other runners, the energy of the crowd, the rush of being in a race—and then they pay the price later by slowing down, depleting their glycogen store, and hitting a wall. I'm constantly analyzing runners' race strategies, and I feel, more often than not, when a runner slows down during the last few miles of the marathon, it's because they didn't practice pacing enough during training. Or there was an unrealistic time goal, and they aimed too high on race day. This is where practice makes perfect. Or as close to perfect as possible. It's through training that you will learn how to run at a particular pace and effort, depending on the distance and workout.

The ultimate goal is to find the perfect marathon pace. To achieve that, you must strike a balance between burning glycogen and burning fat to fuel your run. The best source of fuel for endurance athletes is the fat that is stored in their bodies. Runners need to consume carbohydrates prior to and during their workouts to boost their metabolism just enough to allow the fat-burning process to kick in. When we train at high intensities, we primarily burn glycogen (sugar/carbohydrates), but when we run for long distances at a very low intensity, like in a half-marathon or marathon, our primary source of calories to fuel our muscle contractions is *fat*. It's during those long-distance training runs that your body begins to push aside the carbs for immediate energy demands and starts to free up those fat stores for use during your muscle contractions.

Determining Your Pace

So how do you determine your marathon pace? This is a very important question to ask at the beginning of your training so you know how to set all of your pacing parameters for the next 20 or so weeks. Most beginners have very ambitious time goals that are based on little empirical data to back them up. First, you should take a look at your most recent race finish times. This will help you get a ballpark pace from which to work with. The closer the distance was to a marathon, the better. If you ran a half-marathon recently, go off that time. Take your finish time, multiply it by two, and add a conservative 10 to 15 minutes on to that number. Some coaches will go so far as to add 5 to 7 minutes versus my 10 to 15, so know that my estimate is on the conservative side for first-time marathoners.

Here's an example of how the formula works: If your last half-marathon finish was 2 hours and 15 minutes, double that (4:30), and then add 15 to 20 minutes (4:40 to 4:45 total time, or 10:40 to 10:52 per mile pace). It's that easy! That's a realistic time goal if you follow a marathon-training-specific plan for five to six months.

During your 20-week training plan, I highly encourage you to run a half-marathon race or race simulation workout (one will be prescribed for you during the plan) about 6 to 8 weeks before the full marathon you selected to get a sense of your fitness and current pace.

HEART RATE

Your target heart rate for marathon pace should be at 65 to 70% of your maximum heart rate (MHR). This is an intensity that most runners can sustain for all 26.2 miles. To determine your target heart rate, you first need to figure out what your estimated MHR is. I like to use this formula, from the folks over at *Runner's World*, to get that number:

For runners under the age of 40:
MHR = 208 – (0.7 × your age)

For runners over the age of 40:
MHR = 205 – (0.5 × your age)

For example: A 56-year-old runner would be 205 – (0.5 × 56) = 177 beats per minute (bpm) MHR. Then, their target heart rate at marathon pace would be (177 × .65) to (177 × .70), or 115 to 123 bpm.

While using a heart-rate monitor is the most accurate way to know if you're hitting these numbers, you don't necessarily need one to make it happen. If you want to take your heart rate while you're running and don't have a monitor, simply stop midway through your workout, place two fingers on the carotid artery in your neck, and count your heartbeats for 20 seconds. Multiply that number by three to get your total beats per minute.

Five Smart Pacing Strategies

1. Listen to your gut and trust your body. If you think you're running too fast, chances are you're probably right! If you're breathing heavily and having a hard time hearing your own thoughts or you can't carry on a conversation with a fellow runner, then take those as clear indicators that you're running too fast and should probably slow down.

2. Wear a GPS watch. You'll receive instant, real-time feedback regarding your current pace and distance so you know exactly when to speed up and slow down to hit your goal. Since their debut a couple of decades ago, GPS watches—and the technology behind them—have improved tremendously. Now the feedback is up to 99% accurate.

3. Use a heart-rate monitor. If you want to save a few dollars and purchase a less expensive device than a GPS watch, then get a simple heart-rate monitor. Knowing what your heart rate is while you run can help you better match your effort to your pace and keep your splits steady. The monitors with a chest strap are slightly more accurate than ones you wear on your wrist, but if you don't want to deal with wearing a strap, the wrist-based monitors also work well.

4. Run with a pacer. This could be a friend who has run for a while and consistently clocks the pace you're trying to reach, or a designated pacer in a race who holds a flag with your goal race pace and guides runners, like you, to the finish line just in time.

5. Hit the track. The absolute best way to gauge your training pace is by practicing at a local track. A track is the most valuable piece of equipment that a runner could ask for in terms of pace accuracy. If possible, run the first mile of your next run around a track (four laps) at goal race pace and take note of the effort you exerted to reach it. You are well on your way to grasping what it *feels* like to run at your goal race pace, which is an important skill to learn, even if you can simply glance at your watch to see where you're at.

TYPES OF RUNS

My training philosophy for a marathon includes giving runners a variety of different training runs—short, easy ones, long, aerobic ones, intervals, tempos, and more. Through the use of multiple types of training stimuli, a marathon runner becomes stronger in both endurance and speed. The key is knowing what percentage of specific types of workouts you should prescribe, based on the individual running and the event they're training for. For example, someone training for a 5K will have a high percentage of speed work and a low percentage of slow long runs. And vice versa, a marathon runner will have a high percentage of distance runs and a low percentage of speed work.

Each type of running workout that I prescribe will target a different energy system, stimulating the growth of that system. Each type of workout also trains your muscles differently, either getting them to contract more forcefully, easily, and quickly or to build the strength and endurance required to tackle 26.2 miles. In other words, all of your workouts are necessary and will play an important role in helping you reach that finish line. The goal is to compartmentalize your training, working on developing one energy system at a time.

Your Training Runs

The almighty long run. This is a very important run during the week for a few reasons. First, the long run teaches your body to become resistant to fatigue. It also teaches your body to burn fat as its primary source of fuel while sparing glycogen or muscle sugar in the process. Remember, fat is our best source of lasting energy for marathon running. Second, it's an opportunity for you to practice patience and mental focus for the long haul of a 26.2-mile race, ultimately helping you build resistance to mental fatigue. And third, it simply builds confidence. By logging a few 18-mile runs (and possibly a couple of 20-mile ones) during your marathon buildup, you can look back at your training log in the days leading up to the race and remind yourself of all the work you've already put in and how prepared you actually are.

The marathon-simulation run. This workout is designed to simulate the type of fatigue you will experience during the race itself. It allows you to practice pushing through that fatigue, as you will on race day, and teaches you how to be patient and properly pace yourself over the course of a long run. The last thing you want to do is go out too hard and then hit a wall halfway through. The first segment of this run should be performed at a pace that's about 45 to 60 seconds slower per mile than your goal marathon race pace (GMRP). The second segment is then performed right at GMRP. For example, you will complete 8 miles at an easy pace (45 to 60 seconds slower per mile than GMRP), and then 6 miles right at GMRP, followed by a one-mile cooldown.

Speed work (and I mean that loosely). This doesn't mean that you will be sprinting around a track like Usain Bolt—it just means that you will be running faster and harder than you will during the actual marathon, and possibly faster than you ever have before. Speed work is literally any run that is performed faster than your normal, easy pace. One workout that I like to do is Yasso 800s, named after Bart Yasso, an esteemed member of the running community. He came up with this workout back in the 1990s, but it wasn't until about 10 years later, in 2001, when Amby Burfoot, an editor at *Runner's World* and dear friend of Yasso's, coined the term. Here's how they work: 10 × 800 meters (two laps around a track) with a recovery interval that takes the same amount of time between each. The idea is that whatever your interval times average out to be can help predict your marathon finish time. So, for example, if you run each 800 meters repeat in 4 minutes, taking 4 minutes of recovery between each, then your predicted marathon finish time would be 4 hours. If you average 3:30 for each rep, then your predicted finish time would be 3 hours and 30 minutes.

The easy recovery run. If all of your other workouts are the building blocks of your training foundation, then the easy recovery runs are the mortar. These easy runs simply add mileage and time in the aerobic zone. They are meant to be performed at a pace that is 45 to 60 seconds slower per mile than your GMRP. Elite marathoners sometimes do their easy recovery runs at a pace that's a full two minutes per mile slower than their marathon race pace. Although it's slightly easier to have that big of a discrepancy when your GMRP is five minutes per mile! The easy recovery run sometimes ends with short, relaxed bursts of quick running, or strides. For reference, if you ever watch a track meet on television, you'll see athletes running very quickly up and down the track right before the gun goes off—they are performing strides. These are not all-out sprints, but rather they're very relaxed and controlled sprints that are meant to open up your hips and keep your heart rate up right before a race or workout. These will be prescribed throughout your training plan.

ASK A PRO

RYAN HALL, TWO-TIME OLYMPIAN, AMERICAN RECORD HOLDER, AND 2:04 MARATHONER:

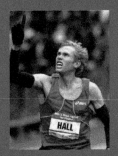

What advice would you give to first-time marathon runners about their form?

Running cues help us run efficiently. The running cues I used while I was running were:

1. I always wanted my forefinger and thumb gently touching as I ran (keeps your arms and shoulders relaxed).

2. I wanted my hands to brush my hips with every swing (keeps your shoulders down and makes sure you move your arms straight forward and back).

3. I tried to relax everything as much as possible.

4. I stayed tall (the taller you make yourself, the easier your breathing will be and the better your body will move.

5. Fast feet! I was always telling myself to pop off the ground (pretending like you are running on hot coals is a great way to do this).

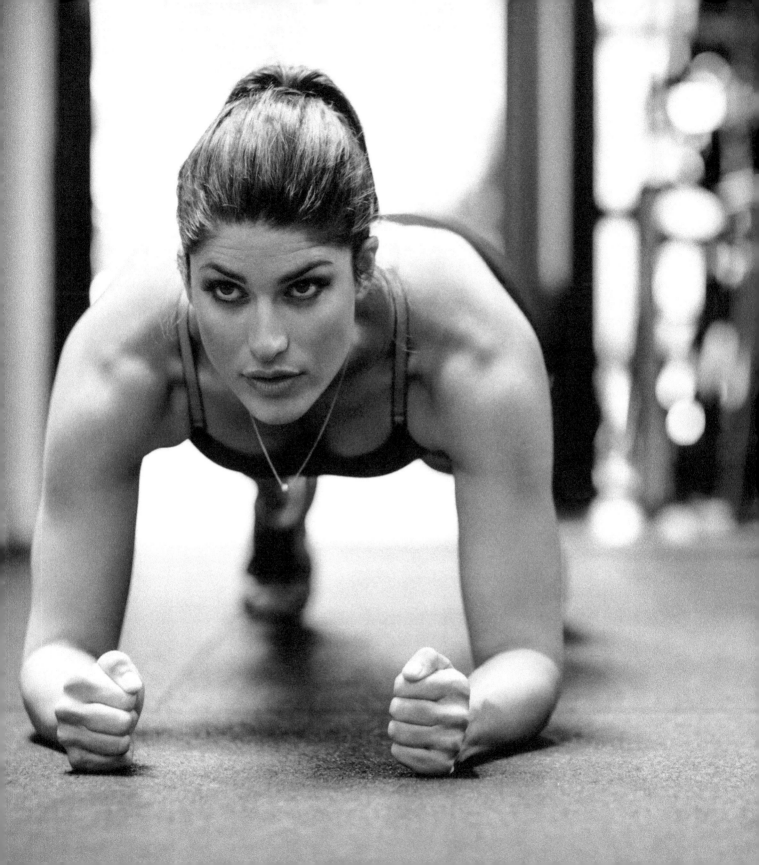

5

STRENGTH TRAINING

When you're training for a marathon, it's easy to get caught up in just logging miles every morning, without giving a second thought about what else you need to do to get your body primed for race day. But it's important to be a bit more well-rounded than "just" a runner. It's better to be a "strong" runner. For best results come race day, you should consider including strength training, stretching, and other types of workouts in your schedule.

In this chapter, we will cover the basics, such as what, how, and when to perform specific exercises that could help enhance your training. These short routines will take just a few minutes and should be completed just a few times per week.

I believe in spreading the workload throughout your week so that nothing feels like it's taking up all your time or energy. Your strength training and stretches will be performed in short increments in between your runs, as you squeeze them in where and whenever possible, and these routines will end up being an integral part of your marathon-training plan in the later weeks of the plan.

WHY WE STRETCH

I'll personally attest to the fact that marathon runners, as a whole, are the least flexible athletes in all of track and field. Typically, the most flexible runners are in fact the hurdlers, which makes perfect sense when you think about it. Marathon runners log mile after mile at an aerobic (slow) pace, keeping their stride length short for a few hours at a time! When muscle tissue breaks down from repetitive pounding, it repairs itself at the length it was last stretched. So when a marathon runner finishes a long training session at a slow aerobic pace, their stride length is about as short as it will ever be while training. The muscle tissue will inevitably repair itself at that length. Compound this phenomenon over weeks, months, and years, and you get short, tight muscles that don't want to lengthen or allow the joints to move freely.

Therefore, stretching before and after your training runs is very important. Marathon runners need to reset the resting length of their muscles after each training run to keep their muscles long and supple. Stretching prior to a workout can increase your stride length and relax tight muscles, thus enhancing your running efficiency, as well.

Stretching is not only great for retaining a muscle's optimal length, but it also encourages recovery. Due to the increased length of a muscle cell after stretching, blood flow is increased to the muscle tissue, which facilitates repair while resting.

During your marathon-training plan, I encourage you to stretch a minimum of four to five times per week, using the routine outlined in this chapter. This will ensure that you are maintaining adequate mobility while piling on the miles in training.

Active Isolated Stretching (AIS)

For almost two decades, I have been using a cutting-edge type of stretching that was developed in the mid-1990s by stretch gurus Phil and Jim Wharton. This father-and-son duo developed a very intuitive way to stretch based on the physiological principles of the nervous system. You may have heard the saying "don't stretch a cold muscle" before. Well, turns out our muscles are always warm enough to stretch, but only the correct way, which means using the nervous system.

This type of stretching, active isolated stretching (AIS), is becoming the new norm when it comes to developing flexibility and mobility in athletes. It uses the nervous system's principle of reciprocal inhibition (when one muscle contracts, its opposing muscle automatically relaxes). To help visualize what I'm talking about, imagine holding a dumbbell and performing a bicep curl. Your brain is telling your bicep to contract to lift the weight up, and through reciprocal inhibition, your nervous system also simultaneously tells your triceps (the opposing muscle group) to relax. This makes the action efficient. The same holds true for stretching. Try this simple stretch: Stand with your knees slightly bent. Lift your right foot off the floor, and grab it with your right hand. Gently pull your foot up to your butt to stretch your quad (the large group of muscles in the front of your leg), hold that for a few seconds, and then squeeze and contract your butt muscles (glutes). You'll notice the intensity of your stretch in the quad increases—that's AIS.

STRETCHES FOR RUNNERS

I've adapted these for you from *The Whartons' Stretch Book*:

Straight-Leg Hamstring

1. Lie on your back. Begin with the knee of the leg you aren't stretching bent and your foot flat on the floor or mat.

2. Take your rope and hold the ends together so that it forms a loop. Place the foot of the leg you're stretching into the loop. Lock that knee so that your leg is extended straight out.

3. From your hip and using your quadriceps, lift your leg as far as you can. Aim your foot toward the ceiling.

4. Grasp the ends of the rope with both hands (to maintain the loop) and "climb" up the rope, hand over hand, as your leg lifts. Keep slight tension on the rope. Use the rope for gentle assistance at the end of the stretch. Do not pull your leg into position or you will irritate the back of your knee.

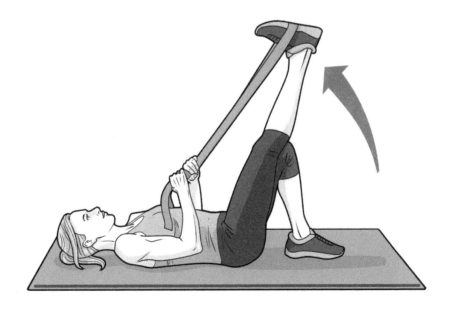

Bent-Knee Hamstring

1. Lie on your back. Begin with one knee bent and foot flat on the floor and bring the other knee close to your chest.

2. Take a rope and hold the ends together so that it forms a loop. Place the foot of the leg you're stretching into the loop. Lift your leg until your thigh is perpendicular to the surface (your knee is at high noon).

3. Grasp the end of the rope with two hands (to maintain the loop). Gradually extend your leg by contracting your quadriceps. This will cause your foot to rise toward the ceiling.

4. The goal is to lock your knee and have your foot at high noon. You may have to lower the angle of your leg from the hip at first. Use the rope for gentle assistance at the end of the stretch. Do not pull your leg into position or you will irritate the back of your knee.

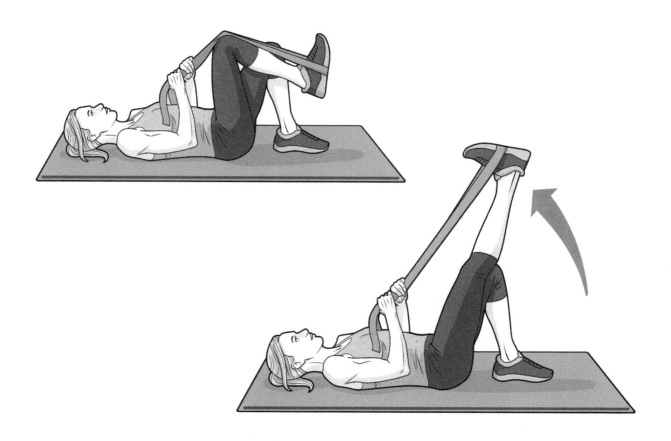

Quadriceps

1. Stand next to a wall for support. Place one hand on the wall and raise your opposing ankle up and grab it with the your free hand.

2. Hold this stretch for 2–3 seconds while at the same time continually contracting your hamstring and glutes on the side you are stretching.

3. Lower your foot down to the ground and repeat.

Gluteals

1. Lie flat on your back, place the outside of your left ankle just above your right knee.

2. Reach behind your right hamstrings and slowly pull both of your legs up toward your chest while using your abdominal muscles and hip flexors to help lift them up.

3. Hold for 2–3 seconds and lower both legs back to the floor or mat; repeat several times.

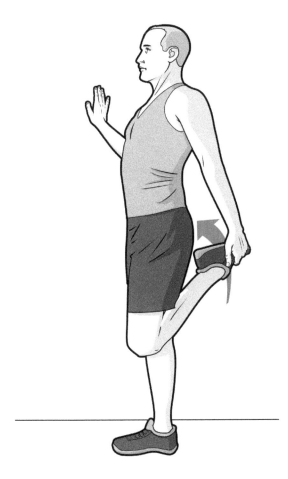

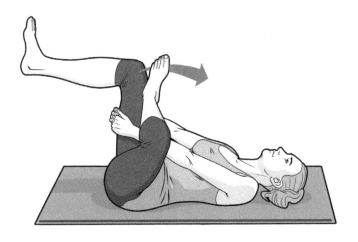

Calves/Gastrocnemius

1. Sit up straight on the floor or mat. Bend both knees with your heels on the floor.

2. Take a rope and hold the ends together so that it forms a loop. Place the foot of the leg you're stretching into the loop. Stretch out that leg into a straight position.

3. Grasp the end of the rope with both hands (to maintain the loop).

4. Activate the shin muscle on the front of your foreleg; this will cause your toes to come toward your body and pull slightly with the rope. Hold this stretch for 2–3 seconds and relax; repeat several times.

THE EXERCISES

When I'm creating training plans, I always try to keep the programming simple. I know that most runners out there only run and very few take the time to perform strength-training exercises either pre- or post-workout. However, I also know that getting them to perform the correct exercises at the optimal time can enhance their performance and help keep their muscles, tendons, and ligaments strong and pliable to stave off injury.

I have selected 10 simple exercises that can be performed in your home (on the floor or standing) and require no equipment, just your own body weight. You'll just be using gravity as resistance. These 10 movements will challenge and improve your strength, power, balance, and coordination.

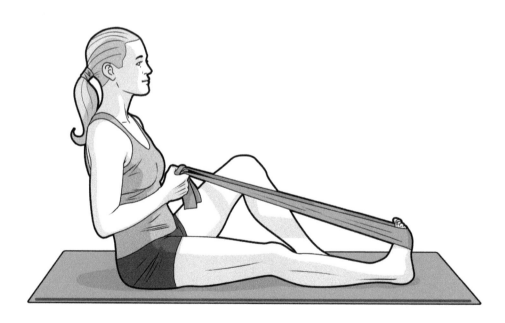

Squat Jump

Stand with your feet shoulder-width apart, arms
by your sides, and then bend your knees to
90 degrees as you lower your hips into a squat.
Keep your abs engaged and jump straight up,
landing softly back in a squat position.

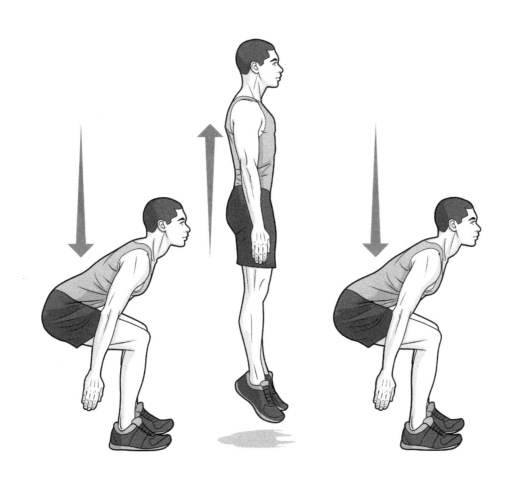

Mountain Climbers

Start in a plank position with your palms on the floor under your shoulders and your legs extended behind you, abs engaged, back flat, and toes tucked under. Bring your left knee in toward your chest, keeping your right leg straight, and tap your toes on the floor. Keeping your hands on the ground, abs tight, and body low to the ground, hop to switch legs, so your right knee is forward and left leg is back. Continue alternating sides for a few reps.

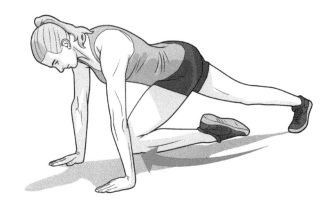

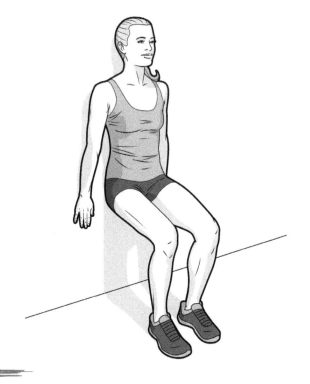

Wall Sit

Brace yourself! Stand with your back against a wall, and then walk your feet forward about 6 to 12 inches. Slowly slide your back down the wall until your thighs are parallel to the ground and knees are bent to 90 degrees. You may have to walk your feet out a few inches to make sure your knees are just above your ankles. Hold this position for 30 to 60 seconds.

Bicycle

Lie faceup on the floor with your knees bent over your hips, your fingers interlaced behind your head, and your elbows out to your sides. Keeping your right knee bent, extend your left leg down toward the floor, as you lift your upper body off the floor and rotate your torso to your right, bringing your left elbow to your right knee. Rotate your torso back through center to your left; switch legs and arms and repeat. Continue alternating, as if you were pedaling a bike.

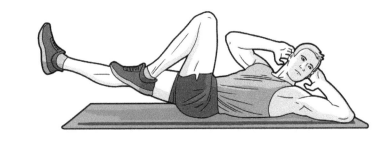

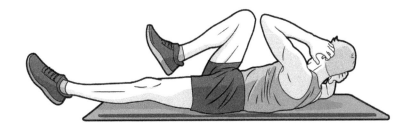

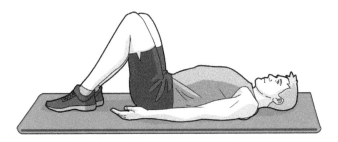

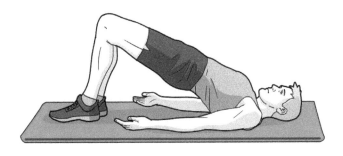

Bridge

Lie faceup on the floor with your knees bent, feet flat on floor, and arms extended by your sides. Slowly lift your hips off the floor, keeping your head, shoulders, and arms down, forming a diagonal line from your knees to your shoulders; hold for a few seconds, and then lower back down to the starting position; repeat.

Superman

Lie facedown on the floor, with your arms extended overhead and your legs extended behind you. Engage your core and keep your shoulders down as you simultaneously lift your arms and legs a few inches off the ground. Hold for one breath, and then gently lower back to start; repeat.

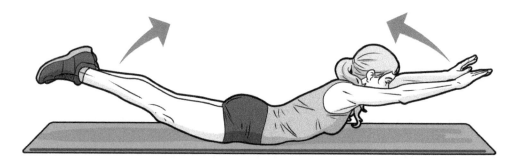

Forearm Plank

Lie facedown on the floor, with your legs extended behind you, your elbows under your shoulders, and your forearms flat on the floor in front of you. Engage your abs and lift your hips off the floor, forming a straight line from your shoulders to your heels. Hold for 30 to 60 seconds, then lower to the starting position.

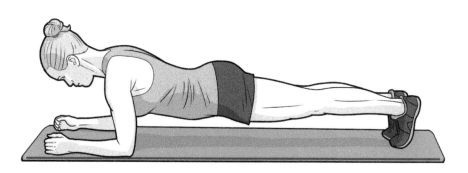

Calf Raises

Find a step along with a handrail to hold on to.
Stand on the step, holding the railing or banister,
and inch your heels off the step's back. Drop your
heels down a couple inches and then come up
onto your toes, making the calf muscles contract.

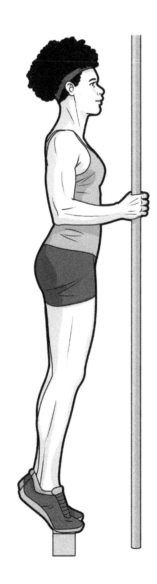
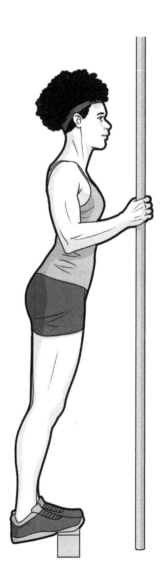

Incline Push-Up

Firmly place your hands on the flat surface of a
low counter or bench, keeping them directly under
your shoulders, and then walk your feet back so
your body forms a diagonal line from heels to
head. Now perform a push-up; repeat.

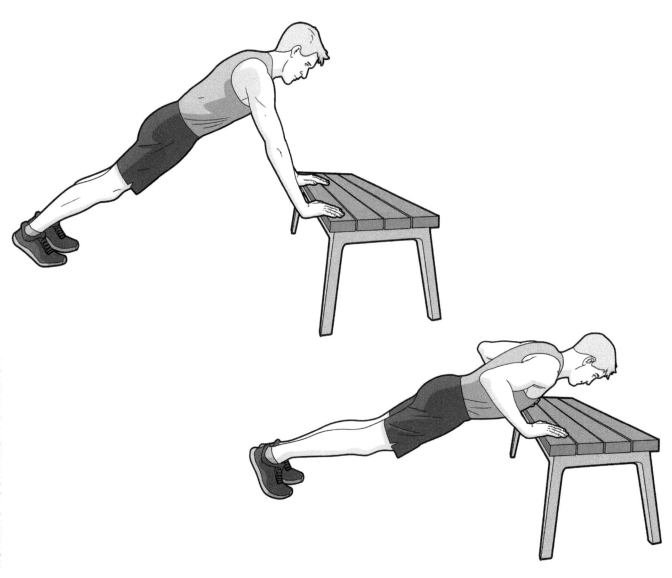

Bear Crawl

Start in a tabletop position, with your palms under your shoulders and your knees under your hips. Lift your knees off the floor, rising up onto your toes, and then slowly "walk" forward with your right arm and left foot, staying low to the ground. Immediately repeat with your left arm and right foot. Stay on your toes and hands, crawling in a straight line, for a few strides.

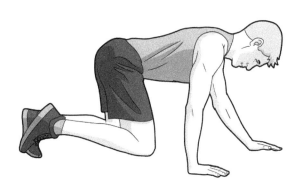 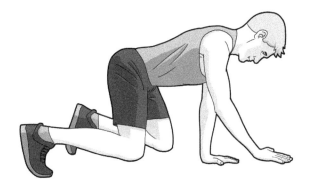

WORKOUTS FOR RUNNERS

I have created five fun workouts that are quick and easy to perform throughout your marathon-training plan. These workouts each have different functions: developing strength, core stability, and mobility. They also don't require any equipment, so you can literally do them anytime, anywhere.

Workout 1: Strong Legs

The goal of this workout is to strengthen your legs and your body overall.

MUSCLE GROUPS AFFECTED:
quads, glutes, calves, shoulders, back, and abs

Wall Sit
30 to 60 seconds / 2 sets / 60 seconds recovery

Mountain Climber
5 to 10 reps / 2 sets / 60 seconds recovery

Superman
10 reps / 2 sets / 60 seconds recovery

Incline Push-Up
10 to 20 reps / 2 sets / 60 seconds recovery

Forearm Plank
30 to 60 seconds / 2 sets / 60 seconds recovery

Calf Raises
10 reps / 2 sets / 60 seconds recovery

AIS: Quads
10 each leg

AIS: Calves
10 each leg

Workout 2: Core Activation

The goal of this workout is to include lots of core activation and develop your flexibility.

MUSCLE GROUPS AFFECTED:
quads, glutes, calves, shoulders, back, and abs

Squat Jump
5 to 10 reps / 1 set / 60 seconds recovery

Mountain Climbers
5 to 10 reps / 1 set / 60 seconds recovery

Superman
10 reps / 1 set / 60 seconds recovery

Incline Push-Up
10 to 20 reps / 1 set / 60 seconds recovery

Forearm Plank
30 to 60 seconds / 1 set / 60 seconds recovery

Bear Crawl
20 feet / 1 set / 60 seconds recovery

Bicycle
10 reps / 1 set / 60 seconds recovery

AIS: Gluteals
10 each leg

AIS: Bent-Knee Hamstring
10 each leg

AIS: Straight-Leg Hamstring
10 each leg

AIS: Quads
10 each leg

AIS: Calves
10 each leg

Workout 3: Joint Mobility

The goal of this workout is to develop flexibility and mobility, increasing the range of motion in your joints.

MUSCLE GROUPS AFFECTED:
quads, glutes, and abs

Bear Crawl
20 feet / 2 sets / 60 seconds recovery

Bicycle
10 / 2 sets / 60 seconds recovery

Squat Jump
5 to 10 / 2 sets / 60 seconds recovery

Mountain Climbers
10 each leg / 2 sets / 60 seconds recovery

AIS: Quads
10 each leg

AIS: Gluteals
10 each leg

AIS: Straight-Leg Hamstring
10 each leg

AIS: Calves
10 each leg

AIS: Bent-Knee Hamstring
10 each leg

ASK A PRO

JOSH COX, AMERICAN RECORD HOLDER IN THE 50K AND A FOUR-TIME OLYMPIC MARATHON TRIALS QUALIFIER

If you had to recommend only one exercise for a marathon runner, which one would it be?

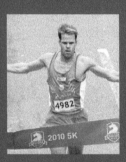

Better core strength makes for a stronger and more durable runner. One exercise I love for developing that strength is the plank. I (almost) always complete this plank circuit (holding each one for 30 to 120 seconds) after my easy runs: First, do a standard plank (palms under your shoulders in a push-up position, with your back flat, legs extended behind you, and toes tucked under). Next, do side planks on both sides. (A side plank is similar to the standard plank, but your body is turned to face one side, with your hips stacked, one hand on the floor, and your other hand reaching toward the sky.) If you're more advanced, you can try lifting your top leg toward the ceiling as you hold as well. Then, do a walking plank: start in standard plank position, but instead of holding still, walk your feet up to meet your hands, pushing your hips toward the ceiling, and then walk your hands forward, back into standard plank position, keeping your arms and legs extended and your back flat throughout. Take five "steps" forward, five steps back, five steps to the left, and five steps to the right.

Workout 4: Even Stronger Legs

The goal of this workout is to develop strength in your legs without excessive movement.

MUSCLE GROUPS AFFECTED:
quads, calves, shoulders, and glutes

Wall Sit
30 to 60 seconds / 2 sets / 60 seconds recovery

Calf Raises
10 / 2 sets / 60 seconds recovery

Incline Push-Up
10 to 20 / 3 / 60 seconds recovery

Bridge
10 to 20 / 2 sets / 60 seconds recovery

Forearm Plank
30 to 60 seconds / 2 sets / 60 seconds recovery

AIS: Quads
10 each leg

AIS: Gluteals
10 each leg

Workout 5: Core Blaster

The goal of this workout is to develop only the core muscles. This workout can be done a few times a week if you like.

MUSCLE GROUPS AFFECTED:
shoulders, all the core muscles, and back

Forearm Plank
30 to 60 seconds / 2 sets / 60 seconds recovery

Bear Crawl
20 feet / 2 sets / 60 seconds recovery

Bridge
10 to 20 / 2 sets / 60 seconds recovery

Bicycle
10 / 2 sets / 60 seconds recovery

Superman
10 / 2 sets / 60 seconds recovery

Mountain Climbers
10 each leg / 2 sets / 60 seconds recovery

AIS: Quads
10 each leg

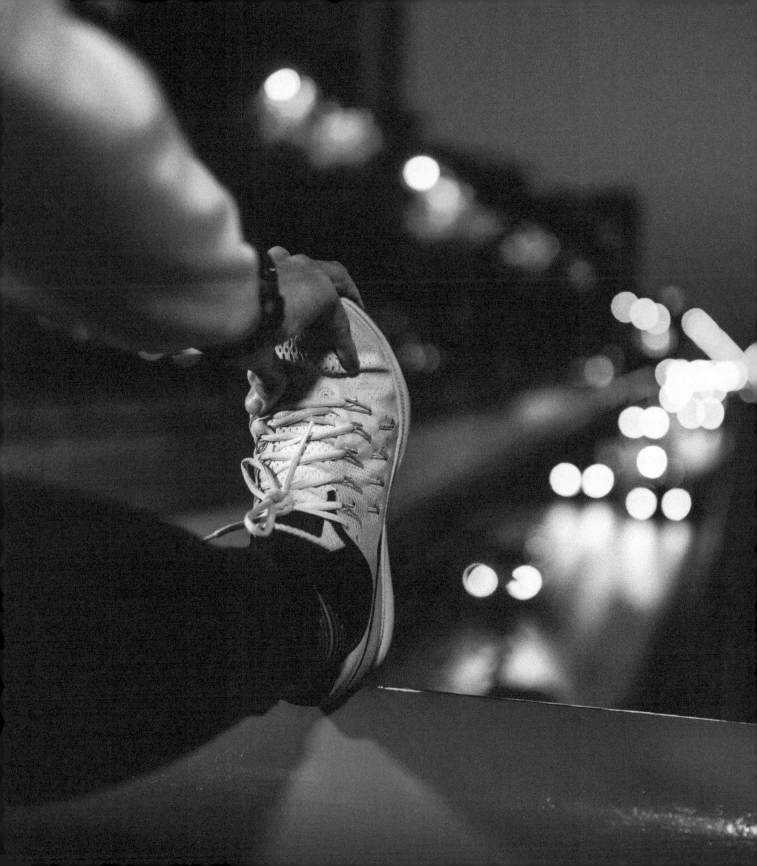

6

SAFETY & INJURIES

'm going to give you the secrets to staying injury-free for your entire running career. Okay, here goes: Sleep well (eight to nine hours each night, with a couple of naps thrown in per week), eat well (get in your fruits, vegetables, and lean meats and drink a ton of water), use common sense when training in risky conditions (i.e., always err on the side of caution when training), adhere to the 10% rule of increasing your mileage each week (the 20-week training program I designed for you will do that), stop training temporarily (for two to three days) if you feel unusual soreness somewhere in your body, and last, but not least, get a massage on a regular basis and stretch regularly. Phew, I think that's everything.

Recovery is key. The best runners in the world know how to push themselves through extreme discomfort and could run hard literally every day if they wanted to, but they don't because they know better. After all, they are the best for a reason. They know how to recover and when to listen to their bodies if anything feels out of sorts. Anyone can go out and run hard every day. But to have the maturity and experience to hold back on your designated recovery days is where the real challenge lies.

This chapter will cover the best practices for safe running, as well as provide tips for preventing, mitigating, and recovering from injuries.

HOW TO RUN SAFELY

As your coach, I don't want you to just run; I want you to run safely. The most significant way to do that is to increase your visibility out on the road, especially if you plan on running early in the morning or late in the evening. To squeeze all of your training runs in, you may have to wake up before your family gets out of bed some mornings or you may have to run after work, and chances are it will be dark outside. If that's the case, make sure you run on a familiar sidewalk or a well-lit road. If neither of those is an option, then consider wearing a small headlamp. There are lots of lightweight, comfortable options out there that you will barely notice are on your head, and the extra visibility is worth every penny. When you're out there with the owls, it's always a good idea to wear a reflective vest so cars and trucks can see you from a safe distance. Wearing anything reflective (apparel, ankle bracelets, buttons, headbands, etc.) is better than nothing.

Always be aware of your surroundings as well. Pay attention to what the weather is doing. Do you see dark clouds up ahead, or is the wind picking up every 10 minutes? Respond accordingly and smartly.

Try to research running-friendly areas if you're logging miles somewhere new. Make sure someone knows where you are, and bring your phone with you in case you get turned around. Or if you're tackling a new trail (fun!), then either run with someone who knows the way or pick up a map before you go so you don't have to worry about getting lost. Whatever the scenario, if something is new to you and you've never experienced it before, then I trust you to use good judgment and common sense.

The longer I coach and the more athletes I work with, the more I realize that the best ones always seem to have the most common sense. Good, sound, common sense seems to go a long way for the top athletes in the sport, who are the ones still running well into their thirties, forties, fifties, and beyond. Why do I mention this? Well, being smart and patient while running in risky conditions—or opting not to run in risky conditions at all—could really help keep an athlete healthy. Some examples of very common conditions that require an extra dose of common sense include running on very rough and rocky terrain; running in the dark; running on the side of a country road with no sidewalks and lots of traffic to dodge; running in the rain, snow, or heat; or running in an unfamiliar place.

Our team is always running on dirt roads, and a few times a week, we run right by herds of cattle. Where the roads and the cattle meet, there are cattle guards that are staked in the ground, are 8 feet long, 20 feet wide, and 2 feet deep, and are covered by metal slats that are about 6 inches apart. These guards pose no threat to cars or bikes; however, runners and cows have a difficult time crossing over them. I guess that's the point, really. But over the years, I have seen runners find a variety of ways to navigate this cattle-restricted area and learned a lot. I have seen runners jump and clear the entire guard while training with the team. I have seen athletes step over the metal strips, while maintaining their pace. And I have seen (usually from the shorter athletes), runners stop and walk gingerly over the guard, very carefully placing their feet on a few metal strips, taking their time, and being cautious. Point is, there are lots of different, smart ways to overcome any obstacles you may encounter on your run. The things that all of the successful solutions have in common though, are, once again, a little common sense and extra caution.

AVOIDING INJURIES

I've been running for 25 years, and it has taken me most of that time to learn how to listen to my body. Runners are notorious for ignoring little sore spots while they are preparing for a big race or event, convincing themselves that an Achilles, a hamstring, or a calf will loosen up after they start running for a few minutes. But it's best to pay attention to your body and adjust your schedule as needed. For example, if I woke up the morning after a tough track session and felt like my right heel was sore, rather than powering through that day's scheduled workout, I'd baby it and take the day off to allow the inflammation to settle down and clear out.

Since moving to California, I have had the privilege of working with a two-time Olympian in Nordic skiing, Nancy Fiddler. She is well into her sixties now, but she still comes out to our weekly track club workouts. I have shared many miles with Nancy over the years, filled with many thought-provoking conversations about training methodology and coaching (she coaches the youth Nordic ski team here). She often talks about her concern for the youngsters who train through all of their little aches and pains, which, as we all know, can eventually lead to big aches and pains that require large chunks of time off later. We chat about how taking one day off this week

if we feel like something's not right, rather than begrudgingly pushing through the discomfort, can prevent us from taking three to four days off the following week.

One thing to remind yourself of regularly is that there's an accumulative adaptation process to training, meaning that you are the sum of all the running that you've ever done in your lifetime. And missing one or two easy runs here and there will not make or break your season—or race.

THE MOST COMMON RUNNING INJURIES

I've compiled a list of the 15 most common running injuries and how best to avoid them.

1. ANKLE SPRAINS: Rolling your ankle is an all too easy thing to do, especially if you're running on rocky, rooted trails. The best way to avoid this injury is to increase your mobility by putting your ankles through their full range of motion before every workout: Point one foot downward, and then keeping your toes on the ground, roll your ankle to the outside and then to the inside, slowly stretching all of the tissues that surround the joint. Switch sides and repeat. This will help loosen up and prep your ankles for the run ahead. If you do happen to sprain your ankle, then rest, along with cold therapy (page 67), is needed.

2. ACHILLES TENDINITIS: This is one of the most common overuse injuries seen among runners. Achilles tendonitis is essentially inflammation of the thick tendon that attaches at the base of your heel, or calcaneus. One cause is tight calf muscles, which results in repeated micro-tears to the structure itself. It takes a while to get to this point of the injury, after running for weeks with a sore Achilles. The best way to avoid this is to stay hydrated through training and stretch your calf muscles frequently (see the calf stretch on page 46). Recovery can take a few weeks if you don't address this injury right away. Also, use caution with cryotherapy or cold therapy, as the Achilles tendon is sensitive to cold and lacks sufficient blood supply to warrant such a modality.

3. BLACK TOENAILS: Your feet actually lengthen when you're marathon training. If you currently train in a comfortable running shoe, you may want to consider going up one half to one full size in your next pair of shoes. When you run long, like for two to four hours, the muscles in your feet begin to fatigue and swelling can occur, which ultimately increases the length and volume of your feet. If your toes start to bump up against the front of the toe box on your now too-small shoes, then you could end up with sore black toenails. If you do get black toenails, then simply purchase a larger size shoe right away. You can always soak your feet in a bucket of cold water to alleviate the discomfort on the tips of your toes as well.

4. BLISTERS: Friction between the skin of the foot and the inner lining of the shoe will cause the skin to weaken and break open. While the blister itself may not mechanically affect your stride, the pain from it can alter your stride mechanics and cause you to unconsciously change your running style, potentially leading to another injury.

The best way to prevent a blister from forming is to invest in a few pairs of specifically designed running socks, ones with two layers of protective material or thicker material that prevent against excessive rubbing. If a blister occurs, stop, take off your shoes and socks, clean the affected site, apply a little antibacterial cream to the area, and cover it with a bandage. Wait a couple of days for the skin to regenerate, then resume running again.

5. CHAFING: When we say "feel the burn," this is not exactly what we're talking about. Chafing, or when your skin rubs uncomfortably against itself or clothing, can occur anywhere, really, but is most common under your armpits and between your thighs. The best way to prevent this from happening is to rub a little Vaseline or a special anti-chafe powder on any potential hot spots before you start your run. Wearing seamless apparel or longer tights rather than shorts will also help prevent this from becoming a problem on your runs.

6. ILIOTIBIAL (IT) BAND FRICTION SYNDROME: When you feel pain on the outside of your knee, this is often the culprit. Discomfort is especially noticeable when you land on the foot of your affected knee. The IT band is a large band of tendon that stretches from the outside of your pelvis to the outside of your knee, and it is used to support and guide your knee as you walk or run. Sometimes the muscle that controls the IT band tightens up and pulls on the attachment point on the bone just below your knee joint. Rolling out the lateral side of your quads with a foam roller regularly (before or after running) can help stretch this tendon out. Rest and cold therapy are recommended for healing.

7. PLANTAR FASCIITIS: I could write four chapters on this injury, but I'll keep it short. Plantar fasciitis is inflammation that causes pain under your heel due to a tight foot arch and calf muscles. The discomfort is usually felt most strongly in the morning when you first step out of bed. As soon as you start to feel pain when you get out of bed in the morning, I recommend following this protocol: Before getting up, stretch your calves by activating the shin muscles (pull your toes up toward your heart, keeping your heel on the ground; and hold for a few breaths). Then slip on your running shoes before you start walking around. Being barefoot can actually stretch your fascia more, which makes the issue even worse. Head directly to the kitchen and drink 8 to 12 ounces of water. Finally, 10 to 20 minutes before you run, stretch your calves (see the calf stretch on page 46). Post-run, use cold therapy directly on the heel to reduce inflammation, and use a baseball or tennis ball to roll out the muscles in your arch for a few minutes.

8. RUNNER'S KNEE: Otherwise known as patellofemoral pain syndrome (PFPS), there's a reason this is now commonly referred to as "runner's knee." You guessed it—there's a high percentage of runners who suffer from it. Basically, this injury creates pain on the front of your knee where the kneecap tracks along a groove. It is caused by excessive friction due to the kneecap being out of alignment, due in part to tight quadricep muscles. Simple quad stretches (see page 45) will help alleviate the tension. For

recovery purposes, take a few days off to allow the inflammation to subside and use cold therapy.

9. SHIN SPLINTS: Typically shin splints are felt in the front part of your leg, below the knee and just above the medial malleolus (inside your ankle bone). Pain and irritation in this area is most often caused by increasing your mileage too quickly or a lack of adequate support in your running shoes. Here's the fix: At the very first moment you feel soreness here, stop running for a couple of days, buy new shoes (ones with plenty of medial support), and begin cold therapy right away.

10. SIDE STITCH: This is not so much an injury as much as it is simply a detriment to your performance. Most people can run, albeit slowly, through a side stitch. What is it? This annoying distraction is a cramping of your muscle tissue usually on one side of the abdomen. When running at high intensities, blood is diverted away from organs that are not contributing to locomotion (the digestive organs, in particular). When there's food in your stomach that still needs to be digested, it competes with the rest of your body for blood supply. This is why a side stitch may occur when you're running on a semi-full (or full) stomach. After your pre-workout (or race) meal, give your stomach time—at least 60 minutes—to digest and empty its contents into the intestine before running.

11. STRESS FRACTURE: Our bones are sturdy, until we overstimulate them with repeated impact forces. The strength of a bone has a direct correlation to a healthy diet—one that's rich in calcium, phosphorus, and vitamin D—and how much stress is applied to the bone itself. Sometimes the correct balance gets out of whack, and a hairline fracture occurs in a bone in your foot or a long bone in your leg. It takes, depending on your age, approximately 6 to 10 weeks for a bone to heal from a stress fracture. Performing non-weight-bearing exercises is the only recovery option, no two ways about it.

12. MUSCLE STRAIN: A muscle strain, not to be confused with a tendon or ligament sprain, occurs when the muscle suffers a small tear. Running quickly or abrupt sprinting is usually the culprit. This broad-range type of injury can heal relatively quickly, since your muscle tissue is very vascular, meaning that it has a rich blood supply, unlike your tendons and ligaments. Cold therapy is encouraged with a muscle strain, and running is advised only when the soreness has completely vanished.

13. HIP BURSITIS: Anything with an *itis* at the end of it denotes inflammation. A bursa sac is the pouch of fluid that rests between a bone and a tendon that may rub over that bone's edge. Sometimes this sac can get inflamed due to excessive rubbing of the IT band (there's that pesky tendon again). The best thing to do to heal is to foam roll the outside of your quad and apply cold therapy to the area experiencing pain.

14. PATELLAR TENDONITIS: Yet another *itis*, this inflammation-based injury occurs at the point just below your kneecap. This is typically an overuse injury caused by the repetitive pounding that occurs when you run. Tight quads are the culprit here, and stretching them out can help alleviate your pain or discomfort. Take a few days off while using cold therapy and focus on stretching your quad muscles:

You will get back on the trails (or road) in no time. If your budget allows, set up a sports massage, and be sure to tell your massage therapist where your pain is so they can home in on that area.

15. BACK PAIN: With all the pounding your body suffers during marathon training, the logging of mile after mile, your back all too often takes a beating in the process. Vertebral disc compression can be a concern for marathon runners. Because of this, I have all of our elite runners (those running 100-plus miles per week) hang from a pull-up bar a few times per week to help lengthen their spines. Creating space between your intervertebral discs helps with the conduction of neural impulses that exit the spinal column, which means that your brain can converse with your muscles a bit better as a result.

Please note that even though I've provided generalized advice for each injury, it's always best to consult with your physician when any "out of the norm" pain arises. They will be able to advise you on your personal path to recovery and healing. Once you have discussed a plan with your doctor to return to training, then you can begin to ease your way back from injury slowly and easily.

RECOVERING FROM INJURIES

Injuries happen! They are inevitable in life, and there's a natural risk that comes with subjecting your body to intense training and massive amounts of physical work (e.g., marathon training).

Training with an Injury

Returning to training can be a challenge not only for your body, but also for your mind. Injuries can cause a major blow to your confidence. Understandably, no one wants to fall behind in their training, which is why it's so important to be flexible with the training and redefine a new marathon goal for yourself, if necessary. It's time to be real with yourself. If the injury occurred close to the marathon race date and you feel that you missed too much training, then it would probably be wise to delay your first marathon for a few months to allow for a proper buildup and, ultimately, much better results.

In Meb Keflezighi's book *Meb for Mortals*, he talks about staying fit while trying to heal an injury. Here's his advice for maintaining your aerobic fitness while recovering from an injury: "Use an ElliptiGo, elliptical machine at a gym, bike (regular or stationary indoor), or do some water running. These are the best ways to keep your running fitness when you're injured." ElliptiGo comes the closest to simulating the running motion, but not everyone has access to one of these specialized machines, so a bike will do just fine to get you moving and outside, where you can enjoy the scenery and feel the breeze on your face.

When an injury strikes, I encourage you to incorporate the workouts in chapter 5 into your daily routine if they do not irritate the injured area. By performing these resistance exercises and stretches, you'll maintain your strength and flexibility for when you do resume training.

Sometimes your training plan misses the mark (starting with too much activity too soon, for example), and sometimes the athlete misses the mark (not recovering properly between workouts or not really listening to their body, for example).

Most running injuries are not severe, or at least they shouldn't be if they are addressed right away and your training is paused accordingly. An athlete can recover very quickly from an injury if it's caught and recognized immediately and then acted on swiftly.

It's estimated that 50% of all runners develop an injury each year, and that 25% of all runners are classified as currently suffering from an injury. Most of these are considered overuse injuries, meaning they develop over time and are caused by running too many miles without ample recovery built in.

BE PATIENT

Marathon runners are highly motivated athletes, in general, and usually have high pain tolerances. They're always tempted to hop right back in where they left off with their training, despite an injury and all its setbacks. But once the pain has subsided, a full range of motion has been restored in all your joints, and there's no noticeable swelling in the area, it is okay for you to consider resuming your training. This return should be a mindful, gentle process.

If need be, consider walking as an alternative to running for the first couple of days you feel like going for a run again. The most important thing is that you're back out there doing it. And when that first training run finally arrives, put on a smile. Venturing out for a run should be an absolute joy. The first week back should be at an easy effort, completing a total distance that's only about 30% of the last full training week you finished before getting sidelined. From there, add 10% each week for about four to six weeks. At that point, if you're still feeling healthy, you can resume full training with prescribed workouts and long runs.

BE GOOD TO YOUR BODY

I always advise runners to pamper and take special care of themselves during marathon training. Doing little things throughout the day to make yourself feel better, more rested, and recovered can help make training easier and enjoyable. Sit down at every opportunity you get; get off your feet and allow your legs to rest when you're not training.

Great Ways to Pamper Yourself for Better Results

Get at least eight hours of sleep every night. While we sleep, our bodies produce hormones that work overtime to repair themselves from the stress of training and life. When we don't get enough sleep, our bodies produce hormones, like cortisol, that can cause negative effects instead. Marathon runners are stressing each of their bodily systems, exhausting their energy reserves, depleting their growth hormones, and damaging tissues on a regular basis. This is above and beyond the "normal" daily activities of other folks. One or two 20- to 40-minute naps a week help with the recovery process.

Apply the rule of RICE periodically. RICE is a mnemonic for Rest, Ice, Compression, and Elevation. The rules are simple to follow for treating a soft-tissue injury, such as a sprained ankle or a strained calf.

Rest. Take a day or two off when soreness is first felt.

Apply ice to the area that's sore for about 10 to 12 minutes at a time, and be sure to wait one hour before applying ice again.

Practice compression. With an elastic bandage, wrap the injury firmly, but loose enough to permit free motion. This reduces swelling and promotes blood flow.

Elevate your injured area above the heart for 15 to 20 minutes, several times a day, to help reduce swelling.

Try cryotherapy, or soaking in cold baths, as a great way to recover from a hard workout or long run. During the summer months here in Mammoth Lakes, elite runners soak their legs in the local creek to recover from hard training sessions. This reduces inflammation in damaged tissues and speeds up recovery from a hard bout of exercise. When you cool your legs, blood vessels constrict, which slows the swelling process. Once your legs start to warm back up, the blood vessels dilate and allow fresh blood to flood in.

Get a massage (or many)! When my wife was running 130 miles per week at various points during her career, we would make it a point to incorporate 8 to 10 hours of massage therapy into her recovery regimen each week. Now clearly, as a first-time marathoner, you don't need to get a massage every day or week, but once every two to four weeks can work wonders for someone logging 35 to 45 miles every seven days. Massage involves mechanically pushing out the by-products of cellular metabolism and breaking up adhesions, or scar tissue, that have built up in your muscles over time, which then allows your muscles to contract more freely and receive an adequate blood supply.

ASK A PRO

CAROLINE LEFRAK, US OLYMPIC MARATHON TRIALS QUALIFIER AND 2:38 MARATHONER

What's your number one safety tip for first-time marathoners?

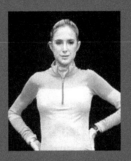

Try to take a day off or cross-train after long or particularly challenging runs. When I first started doing marathons, I would hop on the elliptical with a magazine every Monday after a long run and then go through a quick stretching and core routine. I enjoy the mental and physical break from the mileage, and my legs feel fresher for the next day's workout. Another great substitute is swimming. It gives your lower body a complete rest, and water immersion helps speed recovery. Don't fret about missing a day of mileage. It's always better to be a little undertrained than overtrained on race day.

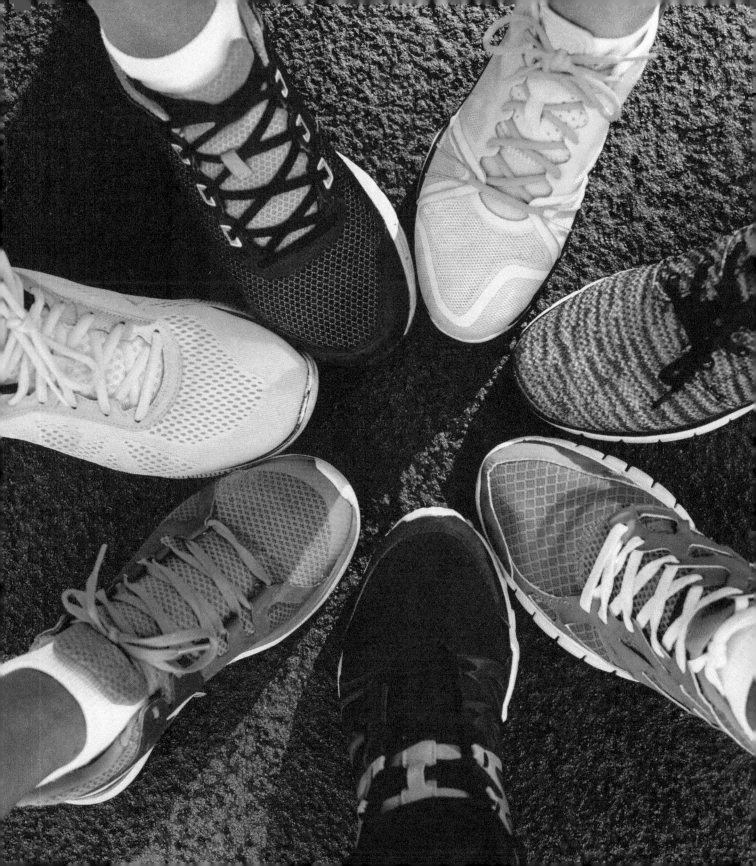

7

YOUR SUPPORT TEAM

**"People often say that motivation doesn't last.
Well, neither does bathing—that's why we recommend it daily."**

—Zig Ziglar

I am often asked how much of running is mental and how much is physical. Well, the answer obviously varies from runner to runner and coach to coach, but my personal belief (along with many others, really) is that training for a marathon is 90% mental and 10% physical. You must be constantly motivated to stick with it, so your brain should be in the game. In other words, you need to be in it to win it. And by "win it," I don't mean crossing the finish line before anyone else. I mean crossing the finish line at all, on your own terms. I work with some of the best distance runners in the country, and they are highly motivated, which makes my job rather simple. I can just guide them along, pointing them in the right direction, versus having to literally knock on their doors at 8 a.m. to convince them to come to practice.

This chapter will begin to peel back the psychological side of marathon training and let you in on what it takes mentally to reach both the start and finish lines of your race.

MOTIVATION

The Internet is filled with motivational quotes and images. I am pretty sure that when you refresh your Instagram, Twitter, or Facebook feeds, you'll notice someone has recently posted a motivational saying or mood-boosting image. Subtle sources of motivation are all around us, we just have to know where to look for them and how to interpret their meanings. For me, personally, the great outdoors is a natural motivator to get out and complete my daily mileage. I enjoy taking in the scenery that surrounds me, especially while running in my hometown, where the granite mountains project up to 13,000 feet.

Watching the athletes I work with train inspires me to keep up my own running and fitness. Even though, I will admit, neither is anywhere close to what it was back in college.

In the late 1990s, I was a competitive college track and cross-country athlete. My event was the mile, or 1,500 meters. I felt like both my body and my mind were designed for this distance, I had good speed, and I could still run 18 to 20 miles, keeping pace with the 10K guys, on Sunday mornings. My goal, as with most college milers, was to break the almighty 4-minute mile. It had been a goal of mine since my very first high school mile race, where I ran 4:56 in the distance. My dorm room was plastered with images of all the great milers, like Roger Bannister, Jim Ryun, and Seb Coe. I had also written little motivational sayings on Post-it notes to remind myself regularly why I was training so hard and was exhausted all of the time. Some of the sayings were, "You are a 3:59 miler," "You are faster than you think," and "You bleed

Green," referring to one of our school colors. While I never broke 4:00 in the mile, I still look back at those days and know that I gave it everything I had, and I ran as fast as I did because of it.

Why am I telling you all this? Because there may come a time when you might not feel like getting up early to slog through a 15-mile run. Or you may not have the energy to drive yourself to the track to do your repeats. Well, these are the moments when you will need to reflect on your goals and why you committed to this journey in the first place. For example, if you're running a marathon for a charity, think about those who will be positively affected by your determination and grit.

SIX EASY WAYS TO GET (AND STAY!) MORE MOTIVATED

1. COMMIT TO SEEKING INSPIRATION ON A DAILY BASIS. Want to make this as easy as possible? Lucky for you, there's an app (or several, actually) for that. Lots of different apps are designed to bring a steady stream of motivation right to your phone. One app sends you motivational videos from great mentors around the world. You could also go old-school and pick up a new book about an inspirational person whom you've always admired. Or you can go real old-school like me and simply write Post-it notes to yourself, reminding yourself of why you're training for this marathon and giving yourself a positive mantra to help fuel you through the miles. Some sample messages could be: "Stronger Today," "A Faster

Me," "Marathon Man," or "I am a Kenyan." I have actually seen that last one on friends' bathroom mirrors. True story.

2. FOCUS ON THE EMOTIONAL REWARD YOU WILL RECEIVE WHEN YOU ACHIEVE YOUR GOAL.

Imagine the satisfaction that you'll get from crossing that finish line, getting high fives from everyone you know afterward, and then hanging that marathon finisher medal (and maybe a race photo) in your office.

3. TRACK YOUR GOALS ON A WEEKLY BASIS.

Being able to see the progress you're making, written down somewhere, will help boost your motivation and confidence throughout your training. During each week of your 20-week training program, you'll have little bite-sized goals to strive for and achieve, like doing a long run that is one to two miles longer than the previous week or completing a run at your GMRP, from which you can judge and gauge your fitness. This steady diet of small obtainable goals will lead to you conquering one large totally badass goal. And hey, even if you fall short of that end goal for whatever reason, know that you were a better person in the pursuit of it anyway.

4. GET A COACH AND JOIN A TEAM.

This person doesn't have to be a professional, just someone who can guide you to a good training plan and then hold you accountable enough to successfully complete it. Most of the world's best runners have personal coaches, individuals who set their training plans and guide them through the plans, not allowing them to deviate from their original goals. (Bonus: You're already ahead of the game with this book, because I'm basically filling this role for you right now.) But along with having a coach, many pros have teammates whom they meet on a semiweekly basis to do group training runs together. These types of people can help hold you accountable throughout your training. Meeting a buddy for a predawn run is much easier than getting out of bed to run by yourself, because now if you don't make it, you're not just letting yourself down, you're also letting down someone else.

5. WELCOME DISTRACTIONS WHEN NEEDED.

To pass the time during your long runs, especially winter "dreadmill" sessions, have a fun distraction at the ready. Many runners use music to motivate themselves during lonely outdoor runs. On windy days when Deena headed out for her second training of the day, she would put her headphones on and blast the Cure or Morrissey to psych herself up for a hilly five-miler. One of my current athletes listens to podcasts or watches the Cooking Channel while he runs on the treadmill, maximizing what he gets out of this time.

6. BE GRATEFUL FOR WHAT YOU'VE GOT.

Sometimes staying motivated while injured is very, very tough. I say be grateful for what you've got. Some of the greatest motivation I can pull from the Internet is seeing people with physical disabilities or those who are facing other challenges conquering 5Ks, 10Ks, and even marathons. If your Achilles is sore, you still have 3,999 tendons that are perfectly fine! Remember that, and then get out there and do something active and productive for yourself and your health. Take this opportunity to set new and exciting goals. When plan A doesn't go according to plan, make a new plan A.

FRIENDS AND FAMILY

My wife and I have always surrounded ourselves with a great team. Some of the finest people in the industry have contributed to our success, including agents, coaches, teammates, training partners, physiologists, psychologists, and strength coaches, among others. We also employ people from outside the running world, professionals in their designated fields, to assist us, including bookkeepers, CPAs, auto mechanics, editors, and anyone else who can help us achieve our goals. You learn quickly in this world that you can't do everything perfectly by yourself without sacrificing something else important along the way. It's all about finding a balance. And being able to depend on a team of people and surrounding yourself with others who also want to see you succeed are two of the best things you could ever do, no matter what you're trying to accomplish. Period.

I encourage you to enlist folks who you can happily add to your power team. Assemble your own Avengers team, like in the Marvel comics, if you will, consisting of superheroes who are close to you and will support your journey to the finish line of a marathon. These are the people who will be in your corner when times get tough, they'll be the ones who rub your feet when they become sore, who meet you at mile 15 of your long run to cheer you on and hand you an electrolyte drink, or simply offer to get you a glass of water or a healthy snack when you need it most. The people who are closest to you can provide a massive amount of much-needed support over the next 20-plus weeks.

By sharing your goals and ambitions with friends and family, you're adding another layer of commitment and accountability to your training goals. Talk about motivation! The more people you tell, the more people you would be letting down by not following through with your training. You can't let others down, especially those who are rooting and cheering for you all the way to the finish line!

Also, know that you will be inspiring others along your marathon-training journey. You may not remember the famous Charles Barkley quote, "I am not a role model." This was a bit controversial for him to say at the time (in the early 1990s), because he was in fact a role model, whether he wanted to be or not. Simply because he excelled on the basketball court, young kids looked up to him and wanted to wear his jersey while they played on asphalt courts around the country. Point is, you may not think you're a role model just because you're training for a marathon, but you are. Those around you will be positively influenced by your passion and your commitment to your goals. This phenomenon can be inversely used by you to perpetuate and sustain your own motivation while training.

With social media, your community can be as vast and broad as you wish. If helpful, enlist the support of friends on Facebook, Twitter, or Instagram. This adds another layer of accountability, plus it usually wins you some extra cheerleaders in the process. Many runners nowadays develop running social support groups to help them through the entire marathon-training process.

I was taught at a young age that those who are successful in and passionate about a specific area of interest constantly maximize the resources that are available to them.

Five Ways Your Crew Can Support You

More often than not, I find that people want to help you through the marathon-training process, but they're not sure how. So I've listed five basic ways that your friends and family members can positively assist you during this time.

1. Have a friend or family member bike alongside you during a long training run. They can offer fun conversation, provide you with water or a sports drink every couple of miles, plus take photos of you that you can post to social media when you're lying on the couch post-run.

2. Hand off the cooking duties. To conserve energy, have a loved one prepare a meal or two for you throughout the week, or ask them to make a takeout run and bring you back something that you're craving to eat. How awesome would it be if you left for your long run at 7 a.m. and a friend, spouse, or loved one greeted you with a nutritious, homemade brunch upon your return? Put them to work!

3. For all you parents out there juggling kiddos and miles on your weekends, ask a friend to watch your little ones in the morning so you can get in your training worry-free.

4. As I've mentioned before, massage therapy is hugely important in your recovery and performance. During the years that I was practicing massage therapy, I found that 80% of the secret behind giving an effective massage was love and the other 20% was knowledge of the muscles and tendons. I encourage you to ask a friend or family member to gently massage your sore feet and legs every now and then. If they're doing this act out of love and trying to help you, then it will be very beneficial to you and your training.

5. Encouraging text messages can go a long way when you're prepping for a race. Let your friends and family know that you would love to hear from them from time to time, especially if they're giving you praise about how proud they are of you.

How Your Crew Can Help on Race Day

Here's a list that can help you direct the support you receive out on the race course.

1. Handing you stuff along the route: If you're planning to consume large quantities of food or gels throughout the race, then your support crew will need to learn the course so they can meet you at strategic points and give you what you need. Note: Receiving assistance along the route is illegal in professional racing, but if you're not vying for the win (age-group or pro), then it usually isn't a big deal. Check the course rules to be sure.

2. Taking photos of you before, during, and after the race for posterity: These pictures will come in handy when you post something to social media, thanking everyone who encouraged you along the way!

3. Holding brightly colored signs so you can see your crew in the crowd: Some of the best race signs that I've ever seen are both encouraging and hilarious. Here are a few of my favorites:

"I THOUGHT YOU SAID 'RUM!'"

"SMILE. REMEMBER YOU PAID FOR THIS."

"ALWAYS GIVE 100%, EXCEPT WHEN GIVING BLOOD."

"MAY THE COURSE BE WITH YOU."

"I BET YOU'RE SECOND-GUESSING THIS NEW YEAR'S RESOLUTION, AREN'T YOU?"

"IT'S A HILL. GET OVER IT."

"FREE BEER AND SEX AT THE FINISH, HURRY UP."

"YOU'RE HOT AND HAVE STAMINA, CALL ME!"

BECOMING PART OF THE COMMUNITY

In the 2000 Olympic Games, the US team only sent one man and one woman to Sydney to compete in the marathon. The marathon—at least at the elite level—was at its lowest point in our country in decades. Just under a year later, professional running teams started popping up all over the place in an attempt to help remedy the dismal state of affairs in US marathon racing. Coach Bob Larson, from UCLA, brought his top runner, Meb Keflezighi, along with Coach Joe Vigil and his star pupil, Deena Drossin (Kastor), and they formed the Mammoth Track Club. They also invited US Olympians from around the country to join them in training at a high altitude.

The goal of forming this team was to emulate what the East Africans were doing: training in large groups and at altitude. During the next Olympic cycle, 2001 to 2004, many runners from around the country and world traveled to Mammoth Lakes for high-altitude training, and by the time the 2004 Athens Olympics rolled around, the United States sent a full marathon squad of three men and three women. Not only did we send a strong squad, but we also ended up getting one man (Meb!) and one woman (Deena!) on the podium. They both came from our small town of 8,000 people, which was quite a proud moment for our community.

I've been part of a team for as long as I can remember: from playing soccer as a five-year-old, to running cross-country and track in high school and college, to coaching our professional team. I can personally attest to the fact that having the support of those around you will play an integral role in your success as a marathoner.

Benefits of Running with a Group

Sharing the workload of your training with members of your team, or even just a single training partner, a couple of times each week will help make the miles fly by (and be way more fun). I don't know if I should use the old saying, "Misery loves company," because *misery* seems a little dramatic here, but I will say that marathoners sure do love company on those hard training days.

Training with a group on a regular basis will help keep you accountable and make you more committed to getting all those miles in. For 26 early Saturday mornings straight, the LA Road Runners (1,000 participants) meet in Venice, California, to prepare as a group for the Los Angeles Marathon. During this half-year training program, friendships and bonds are created over the course of many shared miles along the Southern California coastline.

While in a group setting, it is easy to learn from other runners, many of whom have already completed a marathon and understand the nervousness and trepidation that comes naturally with running 26.2 miles for the first time. Talking with someone who has been through it before is a surefire way to gain confidence about reaching your own finish line.

With the presence of so many running clubs all over the country, gone are the days of the "lonely marathon runner." If you're social, then running clubs are a great way to meet new people who share similar health, fitness, and lifestyle goals.

How to Find a Running Group

How can you surround yourself with a team of positive people throughout your training? I encourage you to link up with a running club or a community of runners in your area. Look online—Facebook and Google searches should point you in the right direction. Many small running clubs offer at least one group training session (usually either a track workout or long run) each week. The next time you head to your local running store for a new pair of shoes, ask if they know of any local training groups or runners who are training for the same race (or one around the same time) as you. It's all about networking.

If you're diving right into marathon training, then you might as well go all in and make some new running friends, both in person and virtually. This will be part of your support crew, your safety net, your posse, the ones who have your back when that little voice in your head tells you to stay in bed on Saturday morning.

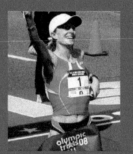

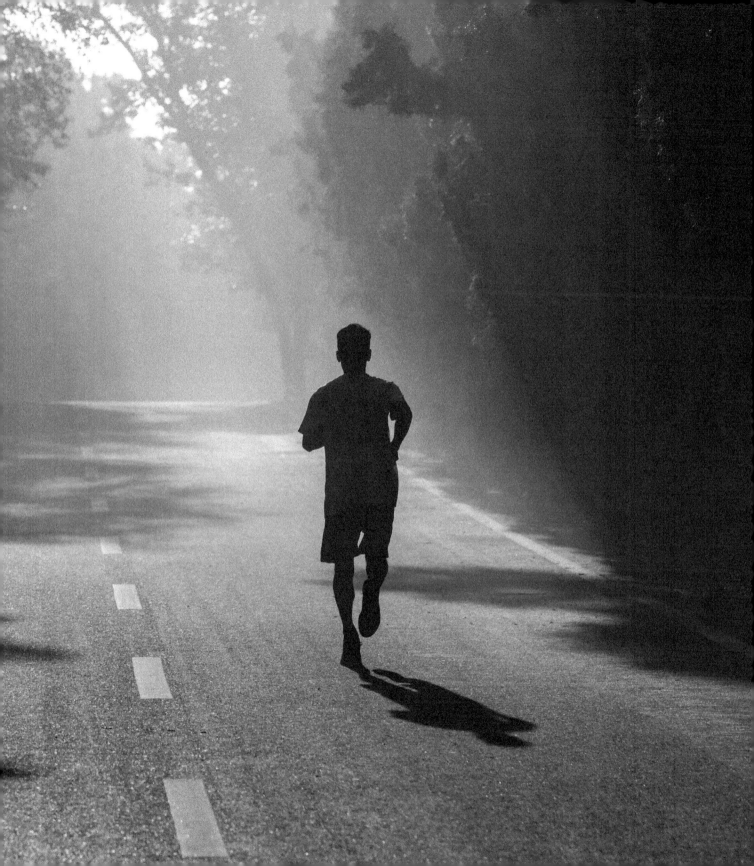

8

THE 20-WEEK MARATHON-TRAINING PLAN

"He who fails to plan is planning to fail."

—Sir Winston Churchill

In this chapter, I will introduce the heart and soul of this book, your official 20-week marathon-training plan. I have pulled together many of the same workouts and ideas that I've given to the thousands of runners who've trained with the LA Road Runners in preparation for the LA Marathon. These workouts are tried and tested, using a combination of both exercise science and experience to construct the perfect plan for you to use on your own 26.2-mile journey.

At the beginning of every week, I will outline each objective training goal that you should aim to meet. I will also provide helpful training tips that will work to maximize your results and up the fun factor throughout your entire marathon-preparation process.

THE PRINCIPLES OF THE PLAN

So how does a coach create a program for the masses? Not knowing who will be reading this book, what your running background is, or what your current fitness level is makes developing a marathon-training program a challenge. So I included only the essential workouts—Yasso 800s (two laps around a track, or approximately half a mile) for speed work; GMRP runs for getting used to running at marathon pace; marathon simulation runs for getting accustomed to running at GMRP toward the end of a longer, steady run; easy aerobic base runs (performed at a pace that's 45 to 60 seconds slower than your GMRP); and the almighty long runs.

To accommodate your varying paces, I have provided a range for your daily goal mileage. For example, the longest run of the training cycle, which comes three weeks before your marathon, has a range of 18 to 20 miles at a pace that's 45 to 60 seconds slower than your GMRP. Some athletes will have a goal pace of 10 minutes per mile for the marathon, whereas others will have a pace of 12 to 13 minutes per mile. It will be your decision as to whether you run the minimum of 18 miles or the maximum of 20 miles. I would suggest that if you are a 12-minute miler, then you should run the shorter distance (18 miles), which will put you out there for about 3 hours and 36 minutes. If you are on the faster side, then I would recommend running all 20 miles (about 3 hours and 20 minutes).

Remember, life happens. People get sick, kids fall ill, work and family obligations have a way of sneaking into an already packed weekly routine, and that's okay. No one workout makes or breaks a marathon-training cycle—it's the total amount of miles you've run and the consistency you've had throughout the whole 20-week training plan that will get you to the starting line healthy and the finish line happy!

The most important part of this training plan is getting in your weekly mileage. If you miss a prescribed speed workout or a GMRP run, don't try to make it up; manage to get in the total mileage of that workout at some other point during the week.

ROOM FOR FLEXIBILITY

Keep in mind that this training plan is simply a guide. Workouts can be shifted around to better accommodate your lifestyle and schedule, if necessary. For example, if it works better for you to do your long runs on Wednesday mornings, then switch them. Your body won't know the difference, and it could make your life (and training) easier.

Strategies for Adjusting Your Schedule

Here are a few strategies to consider when you need to adjust your training plan for any reason during the next five months leading up to your marathon.

1. If you happen to come down with a cold, then take a day or two off, even if it means missing your long run for the week. Rest for a couple of days, get healthy, take one or two easy runs, and then pick back up where you left off—it's that simple!

2. Sometimes runners get injured, but if caught right away, that injury may put you out for only a few days to a week. If this happens to you, be sure to wait until 95% of soreness in the affected area has gone away before you resume training. Then begin with some light training days (i.e., about 30% of the daily running you were doing pre-injury). Once you're back up to full strength, resume training. One important thing to note: When returning from an injury, you should place less emphasis on trying to hit your goal pace times and more emphasis on trying to hit your goal mileage for the day and week.

3. If you find yourself absolutely crushing your workouts mid-plan, feeling great from day to day, then I would recommend you push yourself during the speed sessions (Yasso 800s) rather than the long runs. At some point, you may decide to throw out your initial goal of "just finishing the race" and decide to make your goal "finishing at a certain pace or time" instead. If so, I say *go for it!*

4. Alternatively, if you do sustain an injury and you are knocked out of training for one (or more) weeks, then the most important thing for you to do is to get in the running volume or total mileage at an easy pace after you've recovered. Forget about the goal workout paces; they are not important at this time. Just be consistent with your daily runs and put in the miles, so you can simply finish the marathon.

5. In the unlikely event of your marathon being canceled (it's not very likely but has happened before, as in New York City after Hurricane Sandy in 2012), don't panic. Just know that you've gained a lot of experience and fitness to carry you through to the next one. Also, nearby marathons (ones close in date to your original race) often open their registrations again to let runners affected by the cancellation into their events.

A couple of steadfast principles that you will need to follow throughout your training are 1) adhering to a regular training schedule takes commitment, and 2) you must have the willpower to keep trying your best, get up early on a chilly Sunday morning in January, put on your beanie cap, lace up your training shoes, throw on your running pants, jacket, and gloves, and hit the hard, cold pavement. You must be totally dedicated to achieving your goals, the ones you set out to accomplish on day one of this training plan.

WEEK 1

Use this week to set the tone for your entire 20-week training program. What tone should that be, you ask? Patience. Runners often have this preconceived notion that running should always feel difficult and that they need to push very hard right from the start. But this is simply not the case. Remember, in this first week, if you think you are going too fast, you probably are!

The week starts off (on Monday) with an easy cross-training workout to help boost your metabolism. Tuesday and Wednesday are easy aerobic base runs of two to three miles each, and you should use these to set the tone for the rest of your plan. Thursday is a rest day. Think of your days off as a safeguard against developing an injury, a full day to let your body heal and clear out any inflammation.

Saturday and Sunday have been designed to load up your training week, meaning that both days will carry a bulk of your training mileage throughout the course of this 20-week plan. These two days will be the most critical every week, which is why they both include training runs. I have placed the shorter training runs and "off" days on weekdays, since those are usually your busiest days. Remember, these training runs can be moved around to fit your own personal schedule—just know that you will need to allow time for recovery after each workout, so space them out by adding in one easy aerobic run day between each.

Be sure to start off with a new pair of running shoes this week. It will be important to keep track of the total mileage on them so you'll know when to purchase another pair. This will be especially important in the later stages of training, when your workouts become longer and more intense.

In addition to completing your training runs, remember to do strength work two to three times per week and follow the stretching routine. Performing a stretch session after every run will become increasingly important as your weekly mileage continues to build.

WEEK 1	TYPE OF RUN	MILEAGE	NOTES
M	Cross-Training for 30–45 minutes	N/A	On this cross-training day, focus on furthering the development of your cardiovascular system. The activity you choose should be nonimpact (biking, swimming, using an elliptical, etc.). Keep the effort aerobic and easy (60–70% of max heart rate).
Tu	Aerobic Base Run	2–3 miles	This run is to be performed at a low, aerobic intensity (60–70% of max heart rate), a conversational pace, or 45–60 seconds slower than GMRP. The aerobic base run helps develop a more robust aerobic system, increasing your fat-burning capabilities.
W	Aerobic Base Run	2–3 miles	This run is to be performed at a low, aerobic intensity (60–70% of max heart rate), a conversational pace, or 45–60 seconds slower than GMRP. The aerobic base run helps develop a robust aerobic system, increasing your fat-burning capabilities.
Th	Off Day (complete rest)	N/A	Take this day to allow your body to absorb the training from the first few days. This day will rejuvenate your body for the training week ahead!
F	Off Day/ Cross-Training for 30–45 minutes	N/A	Either take the day off from training or cross-train to further the development of your cardiovascular system. The activity you choose should be nonimpact (biking, swimming, using an elliptical, etc.). Keep the effort aerobic and easy (60–70% of max heart rate).
Sat	Aerobic Base Run	2–3 miles	This run is to be performed at a low, aerobic intensity (60–70% of max heart rate), a conversational pace, or 45–60 seconds slower than GMRP. The aerobic base run helps develop a robust aerobic system, increasing your fat-burning capabilities.
Sun	Aerobic Long Run	5–6 miles	The long run needs to be performed at an easy effort (60–70% of max heart rate), a conversational pace, or 45–60 seconds slower than GMRP.
TOTAL WEEKLY MILEAGE		11–15 miles	A very easy first week of training: You're laying down the foundation for consistency. This is a base-building phase for gradual buildup.

WEEK 2

We are increasing frequency this week, which means I have added one more aerobic base run into your schedule.

Take Monday morning off. Let your body recover from your weekend training. I have given you a range of miles to run every workout. There is no magic number of miles to hit this week, so just try to land somewhere in the middle. If you're a bit tired one day (you are training for a marathon, after all!), aim to do a run at the lower end of the mileage range. The opposite holds true if you're feeling recovered and full of energy—in that case, hit the upper end of the range.

The long run is getting longer. I've added two miles to this run and will continue to add mileage every week for the next four weeks. Simply by adding one extra training run and a couple of miles to your long run, the weekly total mileage increases to about double what it was Week 1. I have mentioned previously in this book that increasing mileage by about 10% from week to week is ideal for staying healthy. Keep in mind that the first few weeks of training are exceptions to the rule since your weekly volume is so low to start. If we were to adhere to the 10% rule in the first four to six weeks, then you would need a 40- to 50-week marathon-training plan to prep yourself for the starting line.

By adding another training run to your week, you are developing consistency with your routine. It will be important to maintain this theme throughout your training. You may be excited, and that excitement may carry into your training, but it's important that you stick to the prescribed paces or efforts listed in the Notes section of each training day.

WEEK 2	TYPE OF RUN	MILEAGE	NOTES
M	Off Day (complete rest)	N/A	Take this day to allow your body to absorb the training from the previous week. This day will rejuvenate your body for the training week ahead!
Tu	Aerobic Base Run	3-4 miles	This run is to be performed at a low, aerobic intensity (60–70% of max heart rate), a conversational pace, or 45–60 seconds slower than GMRP. The aerobic base run helps develop a robust aerobic system, increasing your fat-burning capabilities.
W	Aerobic Base Run	2-3 miles	This run is to be performed at a low, aerobic intensity (60–70% of max heart rate), a conversational pace, or 45–60 seconds slower than GMRP. The aerobic base run helps develop a robust aerobic system, increasing your fat-burning capabilities.
Th	Aerobic Base Run	3-4 miles	This run is to be performed at a low, aerobic intensity (60–70% of max heart rate), a conversational pace, or 45–60 seconds slower than GMRP. The aerobic base run helps develop a robust aerobic system, increasing your fat-burning capabilities.
F	Off Day/ Cross-Training for 30–45 minutes	N/A	Either take the day off from training or cross-train to further the development of your cardiovascular system. The activity you choose should be nonimpact (biking, swimming, using an elliptical, etc.). Keep the effort aerobic and easy (60–70% of max heart rate).
Sat	Aerobic Base Run	2-3 miles	This run is to be performed at a low, aerobic intensity (60–70% of max heart rate), a conversational pace, or 45–60 seconds slower than GMRP. The aerobic base run helps develop a robust aerobic system, increasing your fat-burning capabilities.
Sun	Aerobic Long Run	7-8 miles	The long run should be performed at an easy effort (60–65% of max heart rate), a conversational pace, or 45–60 seconds slower than GMRP. Remember to bring fluids along and take a sip every 15–25 minutes.
TOTAL WEEKLY MILEAGE		17–22 miles	The increase in mileage from Week 1 (11–15 miles) to this week is 46–54%.

WEEK 3

You've probably heard that if you do anything for 21 days, it becomes a habit. Well, whether that's true or not, you are now three weeks into your marathon-training plan, and there is no turning back. Commit to making this a habit!

You are continuing to build your aerobic base, or foundation. This concept was pioneered by the great New Zealand coach Arthur Lydiard back in the 1960s. In his book *Running to the Top*, Lydiard talks about how, when athletes develop their early fitness by running easy, long mileage, they're then better able to handle the rigors of more intense training later in the season. He encourages runners to build their base mileage for "as long as possible." We are taking a similar approach for the first six weeks of your marathon-training plan.

I took the liberty of upping this week's training volume by 13 to 17%, a marginal increase that is getting us closer to the standard 10% increase we'll soon begin making from week to week. We'll continue to add one to two miles to your weekly long run, which is performed at an easy aerobic pace, as well.

During this phase, in which we're building your aerobic base, your body is learning to metabolize fat as a fuel source, something that will come in handy later in your training plan (and could help you get that beach body!).

On Thursday, I will introduce something new, an aerobic base run with short, easy sprints, or "strides," tacked on at the end. These are basically relaxed sprints that help improve your efficiency and your form. Strides also help with stretching out your hips and developing power and quickness in your legs. For best results, perform them on a flat surface.

WEEK 3	TYPE OF RUN	MILEAGE	NOTES
M	Off Day (complete rest)	N/A	Take this day to allow your body to absorb the training from the previous week. This day will rejuvenate your body for the training week ahead!
Tu	Aerobic Base Run	3–4 miles	This run is to be performed at a low, aerobic intensity (60–70% of max heart rate), a conversational pace, or 45–60 seconds slower than GMRP. The aerobic base run helps develop a robust aerobic system, increasing your fat-burning capabilities.
W	Aerobic Base Run	2–3 miles	This run is to be performed at a low, aerobic intensity (60–70% of max heart rate), a conversational pace, or 45–60 seconds slower than GMRP. The aerobic base run helps develop a robust aerobic system, increasing your fat-burning capabilities.
Th	Aerobic Base Run, plus 5× Strides (relaxed sprints)	4–5 miles	Perform your aerobic base run of 4–5 miles. Then find a nice stretch of road with solid footing to perform your strides afterward.
F	Off Day/ Cross-Training for 30–45 minutes	N/A	Either take the day off from training or cross-train to further the development of your cardiovascular system. The activity you choose should be nonimpact (biking, swimming, using an elliptical, etc.). Keep the effort aerobic and easy (60–70% of max heart rate).
Sat	Aerobic Base Run	3–4 miles	This run is to be performed at a low, aerobic intensity (60–70% of max heart rate), a conversational pace, or 45–60 seconds slower than GMRP. The aerobic base run helps develop a robust aerobic system, increasing your fat-burning capabilities.
Sun	Aerobic Long Run	8–9 miles	The long run should be performed at an easy effort (60–65% of max heart rate), a conversational pace, or 45–60 seconds slower than GMRP. Remember to bring fluids along and take a sip every 15–25 minutes.
TOTAL WEEKLY MILEAGE		20–25 miles	The increase in mileage from Week 2 (17–22 miles) to this week is 13–17%.

WEEK 4

So more of the same here, but that doesn't mean it's not still incredibly important! Think of it this way—you're basically banking miles for the marathon. During your 20 weeks of training, you're slowly depositing time and energy (in the form of miles) into a bank account filled with aerobic conditioning. Then, on race morning, you get to make a BIG, one-time withdrawal from the account to complete your marathon.

Keep making those deposits! Every run counts as you grow from week to week. By now, you have been working through, sorting out, and organizing your training schedule to best fit in with your other daily tasks and responsibilities. It's important to have this nailed down by the time you reach the "meat and potatoes" part of your training (Weeks 8 to 17), which will be quite demanding of your time and energy. But with a little patience, you will slowly get there. Remember the old saying, "How do you eat an elephant? One bite at a time." The same holds true for marathon training. Simply replace eat with run, elephant with marathon, and bite with mile.

Your body is becoming accustomed to training five days a week and running back-to-back runs on the weekend. You are slowly developing a callousness to the training. Even when you're tired before a run, you're still able to complete the distance with relative ease. There are many times an athlete has come up to me before a hard workout in the marathon-training buildup and say, "Coach, my legs are so tired, I don't think I can hit the times for today, let alone finish the workout." And then, guess what—they almost always do.

WEEK 4	TYPE OF RUN	MILEAGE	NOTES
M	Off Day (complete rest)	N/A	Take this day to allow your body to absorb the training from the previous week. This day will rejuvenate your body for the training week ahead!
Tu	Aerobic Base Run	4–5 miles	This run is to be performed at a low, aerobic intensity (60–70% of max heart rate), a conversational pace, or 45–60 seconds slower than GMRP. The aerobic base run helps develop a robust aerobic system, increasing your fat-burning capabilities.
W	Aerobic Base Run	3–4 miles	This run is to be performed at a low, aerobic intensity (60–70% of max heart rate), a conversational pace, or 45–60 seconds slower than GMRP. The aerobic base run helps develop a robust aerobic system, increasing your fat-burning capabilities.
Th	Aerobic Base Run, plus 5× Strides (relaxed sprints)	4–5 miles	Perform your easy run of 4–5 miles. Then find a nice stretch of road with solid footing to perform your strides afterward.
F	Off Day/ Cross-Training for 30–45 minutes	N/A	Either take the day off from training or cross-train to further the development of your cardiovascular system. The activity you choose should be nonimpact (biking, swimming, using an elliptical, etc.). Keep the effort aerobic and easy (60–70% of max heart rate).
Sat	Aerobic Base Run	4–5 miles	This run is to be performed at a low, aerobic intensity (60–70% of max heart rate), a conversational pace, or 45–60 seconds slower than GMRP. The aerobic base run helps develop a robust aerobic system, increasing your fat-burning capabilities.
Sun	Aerobic Long Run	9–10 miles	The long run should be performed at an easy effort (60–65% of max heart rate), a conversational pace, or 45–60 seconds slower than GMRP. Remember to bring fluids along and take a sip every 15–25 minutes.
TOTAL WEEKLY MILEAGE		24–29 miles	The increase in mileage from Week 3 (20–25 miles) to this week is 16–20%.

WEEK 5

After this week, you'll be 20% done with your training. Can you believe it?! It's the equivalent of running the first six miles of the marathon. You should be feeling warmed up by now, and well on your way to finding a groove in your training.

Your weekly volume is slowly ticking up by 10 to 12% this week. We are now in the zone of that famous 10% increase per week rule. Your muscles, tendons, and bones are getting stronger and stronger. To help reduce the impact of repetitive pounding on the road, however, I do recommend that you try to perform a few of your training runs on a dirt path or trail each week. If this is not possible, then consider running on the shorter end of my daily mileage recommendations.

Keep in mind that you want to get to your long run feeling as rested as possible, as you're now well into the double digits mileage-wise. Try to dedicate 30 to 60 minutes to your recovery every night this week.

With the slow, aerobic miles really starting to accumulate now, it is important to keep up with your stretching. Aim to stretch three to four times each week after your runs. Your midweek strides will also help to increase your flexibility and stride length.

During this week's long run, be sure to consume the beverage you'll be drinking on race day, sipping four to five ounces every 20 to 30 minutes. Carry a bottle with you and set your watch to beep every 20 to 30 minutes as a reminder to drink your fluids. By consuming fluids with sugar and electrolytes, you will recover faster and be better prepared to get back to work the following week.

This week, you are running more miles than the actual marathon distance! It's an accomplishment worth noting that you should truly be proud of.

WEEK 5	TYPE OF RUN	MILEAGE	NOTES
M	Off Day (complete rest)	N/A	Take this day to allow your body to absorb the training from the previous week. This day will rejuvenate your body for the training week ahead!
Tu	Aerobic Base Run	4–5 miles	This run is to be performed at a low, aerobic intensity (60–70% of max heart rate), a conversational pace, or 45–60 seconds slower than GMRP. The aerobic base run helps develop a robust aerobic system, increasing your fat-burning capabilities.
W	Aerobic Base Run	4–5 miles	This run is to be performed at a low, aerobic intensity (60–70% of max heart rate), a conversational pace, or 45–60 seconds slower than GMRP. The aerobic base run helps develop a robust aerobic system, increasing your fat-burning capabilities.
Th	Aerobic Base Run, plus 5× Strides (relaxed sprints)	4–5 miles	Perform your easy run of 4–5 miles. Then find a nice stretch of road with solid footing to perform your strides afterward.
F	Off Day/ Cross-Training for 30–45 minutes	N/A	Either take the day off from training or cross-train to further the development of your cardiovascular system. The activity you choose should be nonimpact (biking, swimming, using an elliptical, etc.). Keep the effort aerobic and easy (60–70% of max heart rate).
Sat	Aerobic Base Run	4–5 miles	This run is to be performed at a low, aerobic intensity (60–70% of max heart rate), a conversational pace, or 45–60 seconds slower than GMRP. The aerobic base run helps develop a robust aerobic system, increasing your fat-burning capabilities.
Sun	Aerobic Long Run	11–12 miles	The long run should be performed at an easy effort (60–65% of max heart rate), a conversational pace, or 45–60 seconds slower than GMRP. Remember to bring fluids along and take a sip every 15–25 minutes.
TOTAL WEEKLY MILEAGE		27–32 miles	The increase in mileage from week 4 (24–29 miles) to this week is 10–12%.

WEEK 6

At last, a recovery week! It's time to back off from building fitness and give your body (and mind) some time to recover. I have reduced your training volume by 25 to 30% this week. Over the past five weeks, you've already logged between 118 and 147 miles. No, really! Do the math. Again, you want to keep track of the mileage on your running shoes. Once you reach 300 to 350 miles, it's time to get a new pair.

Many of your body's structural adaptations to the training stimulus will be made during this "down" time. Inflammation will get a chance to clear out, and your body will grow stronger and even more ready to tackle your next few weeks of training.

There are many physiological reasons to reduce your mileage and intensity this week, but the mental relaxation that comes with it is a welcome perk as well. This mini-break from training will give you a chance to catch up on work, family time, projects around the house—you name it.

Take advantage of your extra energy this week to be productive, but also keep in mind that you are resting for a reason—the weeks of intense training ahead. If you are participating in any other organized sports or activities, I would suggest scaling back or eliminating them altogether to make more time for your marathon training.

Next week, you will feel lighter on your feet, thanks to the rest you're taking now. Keep with our theme of patience—if you feel good this week, hold back, and save "it" for the upcoming training.

Consider signing up for a short race, maybe a 5K or 10K, in the coming weeks to help keep your competitive juices flowing. If you do enter a race, try to slip your long run into the beginning of the week, swapping it in for an 800-meter workout or GMRP run.

WEEK 6	TYPE OF RUN	MILEAGE	NOTES
M	Off Day (complete rest)	N/A	Take this day to allow your body to absorb the training from the previous week. This day will rejuvenate your body for the training week ahead!
Tu	Aerobic Base Run	3–4 miles	This run is to be performed at a low, aerobic intensity (60–70% of max heart rate), a conversational pace, or 45–60 seconds slower than GMRP. The aerobic base run helps develop a robust aerobic system, increasing your fat-burning capabilities.
W	Aerobic Base Run	3–4 miles	This run is to be performed at a low, aerobic intensity (60–70% of max heart rate), a conversational pace, or 45–60 seconds slower than GMRP. The aerobic base run helps develop a robust aerobic system, increasing your fat-burning capabilities.
Th	Aerobic Base Run, plus 5× Strides (relaxed sprints)	4–5 miles	Perform your easy run of 4–5 miles. Then find a nice stretch of road with solid footing to perform your strides afterward.
F	Off Day/ Cross-Training for 30–45 minutes	N/A	Either take the day off from training or cross-train to further the development of your cardiovascular system. The activity you choose should be nonimpact (biking, swimming, using an elliptical, etc.). Keep the effort aerobic and easy (60–70% of max heart rate).
Sat	Aerobic Base Run	3–4 miles	This run is to be performed at a low, aerobic intensity (60–70% of max heart rate), a conversational pace, or 45–60 seconds slower than GMRP. The aerobic base run helps develop a robust aerobic system, increasing your fat-burning capabilities.
Sun	Aerobic Long Run	6–7 miles	The long run should be performed at an easy effort (60–65% of max heart rate), a conversational pace, or 45–60 seconds slower than GMRP. Remember to bring fluids along and take a sip every 15–25 minutes.
TOTAL WEEKLY MILEAGE		19–24 miles	This is a recovery week, or a reduction week. It's a very easy sixth week of training. The decrease in mileage from Week 5 (27–32 miles) to this week is 25–29%.

WEEK 7

Right back at it! I hope you enjoyed that small reprieve from the rigors of building up your marathon fitness, but now it's time to start building up your strength. For your body to adapt and improve during marathon training, you need a couple of different types of stimulus. They don't have to be overdone; however, they do have to be touched on each week. Two of your workouts this week will do just that. I have increased your training volume by only 3 to 11%, and the stimulus lies within your harder training sessions.

Workout 1, scheduled for Thursday, is a short-and-sweet speed session that can be performed on a track or on the road (the distance needs to be measured). Let this be your introduction to the Yasso 800s. Start off with a one-mile warm-up, running easy, and then stretch for a few minutes. When you feel ready, run your first interval (two laps on a track, or ½ mile) at your GMRP.

Take a recovery interval that's the same length of time as your hard effort was. Cool down with a one-mile easy run. This is the first of five Yasso 800s workouts, so be patient with your times. Start off slowly and work your way into it. Be sure to write down your interval times—you'll use them as benchmarks for future workouts later.

Workout 2, scheduled for Sunday, takes a different approach to your typical long run. The total distance is 11 miles, but you'll perform the first six miles at a slow, easy aerobic pace, and then follow it with four miles at your GMRP. Be sure to add on an easy, one-mile cooldown run at the end.

Always keep in mind that you need to run at a very easy pace, giving you an active recovery, on the days in between the two harder sessions. You will need to make sure that the days you run the aerobic base runs, you should keep it at a very easy effort. This will allow you to recover from the workouts and rest up for the marathon-simulation run on Sunday. The increase in mileage from Week 5 (27–32 miles) to this week is 3–11%.

WEEK 7	TYPE OF RUN	MILEAGE	NOTES
M	Off Day (complete rest)	N/A	Take this day to allow your body to absorb the training from the previous week. This day will rejuvenate your body for the training week ahead!
Tu	Aerobic Base Run	5–6 miles	This run is to be performed at a low, aerobic intensity (60–70% of max heart rate), a conversational pace, or 45–60 seconds slower than GMRP. The aerobic base run helps develop a robust aerobic system, increasing your fat-burning capabilities.
W	Aerobic Base Run, plus 5× Strides (relaxed sprints)	5–6 miles	Perform your easy run of 5–6 miles. Then find a nice stretch of road with solid footing to perform your strides afterward.
Th	Warm-Up: 1-mile easy run Main Set: 4 × 800m @ GMRP, with equal recovery Cooldown: 1-mile easy run	4 miles	Start with a 1-mile easy warm-up run, take 5 minutes to stretch, and then start the main set. Take a walking recovery interval after each rep of equal time as your 800m interval (e.g., if 800m = 4:30, then your recovery is 4:30). End with a 1-mile easy cooldown run.
F	Off Day/Cross-Training for 30–45 minutes	N/A	Either take the day off from training or cross-train to further the development of your cardiovascular system. The activity you choose should be non-impact (biking, swimming, using an elliptical, etc.). Keep the effort aerobic and easy (60–70% of max heart rate).
Sat	Aerobic Base Run	5–6 miles	This run is to be performed at a low, aerobic intensity (60–70% of max heart rate), a conversational pace, or 45–60 seconds slower than GMRP. The aerobic base run helps develop a robust aerobic system, increasing your fat-burning capabilities.
Sun	Marathon Simulation Run: 6 miles at 45–60 seconds slower per mile than GMRP, then 4 miles at GMRP, and 1-mile easy cooldown run	11 miles	Start the first 6 miles at 45–60 seconds slower per mile than GMRP. Then run 4 miles at GMRP, and finish with a 1-mile easy cooldown run.
TOTAL WEEKLY MILEAGE		30–33 miles	You're starting workouts this week!

WEEK 8

Stick with taking your rest day on Monday. You need this day to recover and absorb your training from the weekend. This week ends up being only 6 to 9% more total mileage than last week, but your emphasis will be on the long run, as it climbs to 13 to 14 miles at an easy, aerobic effort.

You are going up in mileage this week, with a GMRP run scheduled for Thursday. The aim of this workout is to get into a groove and figure out your pacing strategy for the race. This pace should still feel comfortable and allow you to run relaxed, with good posture and form.

They say that repetition is the mother of all learning, and if this is indeed the case, then running at GMRP about once a week is the best way to get a feel for your marathon effort, cadence, and pace. You are not only training the muscles and heart for the marathon, but you're also training the nervous system to contract and direct your muscles, refining their capabilities.

Sunday's long run should be at or just longer than a half-marathon distance (13.1 miles). You're halfway home! Your pace should still be easy and comfortable (45 to 60 seconds slower than GMRP). Try to perform this run on a dirt road or trail to help cushion the repetitive impact forces of your landing.

If you are doing some cross-training during the week, try to keep it at a low intensity and aerobic. I have plugged this option in to help your metabolism, while eliminating excessive pounding on your joints. It's completely up to you whether you incorporate this type of activity into your routine.

WEEK 8	TYPE OF RUN	MILEAGE	NOTES
M	Off Day (complete rest)	N/A	Take this day to allow your body to absorb the training from the previous week. This day will rejuvenate your body for the training week ahead!
Tu	Aerobic Base Run	4–5 miles	This run is to be performed at a low, aerobic intensity (60–70% of max heart rate), a conversational pace, or 45–60 seconds slower than GMRP. The aerobic base run helps develop a robust aerobic system, increasing your fat-burning capabilities.
W	Aerobic Base Run, plus 5× Strides (relaxed sprints)	4–5 miles	Perform your easy run of 4–5 miles. Then find a nice stretch of road with solid footing to perform your strides afterward.
Th	Warm-Up: 1-mile easy run Main Set: 4 miles at GMRP Cooldown: 1-mile easy run	6 miles	Start with a 1-mile easy warm-up run, take 5 minutes to stretch, then start the main set. Run 4 miles at GMRP. End with a 1-mile easy cooldown run.
F	Off Day/ Cross-Training for 30–45 minutes	N/A	Either take the day off from training or cross-train to further the development of your cardiovascular system. The activity you choose should be nonimpact (biking, swimming, using an elliptical, etc.). Keep the effort aerobic and easy (60–70% of max heart rate).
Sat	Aerobic Base Run	5–6 miles	This run is to be performed at a low, aerobic intensity (60–70% of max heart rate), a conversational pace, or 45–60 seconds slower than GMRP. The aerobic base run helps develop a robust aerobic system, increasing your fat-burning capabilities.
Sun	Aerobic Long Run	13–14 miles	The long run should be performed at an easy effort (60–65% of max heart rate), a conversational pace, or 45–60 seconds slower than GMRP. Remember to bring fluids along and take a sip every 15–25 minutes.
TOTAL WEEKLY MILEAGE		32–36 miles	You are adding a good chunk of mileage in Week 8. The increase in mileage from Week 7 (30–33 miles) to this week is 6–9%.

WEEK 9

This is another recovery week! Your volume is reduced by 25 to 29% to help freshen up your legs. If you haven't been doing the cross-training, this might be a great week to try swimming, cycling, or an elliptical machine as an alternative to taking an off day. This approach will help supplement your overall aerobic fitness.

Performing strides after your aerobic base run is still very important. Be sure to include those in your workout, as they will help maintain your quick turnover and stride length from week to week.

Nine weeks in—it's time for a massage. Pamper yourself! Look at the expense as an investment, an insurance policy that will help you get to the starting line healthy. Don't let another few months go by without one. And while you're there, go ahead and schedule appointments for later down the road, maybe at Weeks 12 and 15.

Be sure to keep up with your weight training and stretching routine this week. That should be a constant throughout your training from week to week, even though they vary in intensity and volume. Keeping your muscles stimulated through resistance work will help maintain balance in tone and symmetry between your right and left sides, which is important for staying healthy and injury-free.

If training is starting to feel monotonous, mix things up! Try running in a different place or with someone new. Since your Sunday run is much shorter this week, use that "extra" time to drive to a new trail or to meet a friend for coffee afterward. Be creative this week, knowing you may have a few more minutes every morning. This little change could help rejuvenate your spirits and enhance your mood.

WEEK 9	TYPE OF RUN	MILEAGE	NOTES
M	Off Day (complete rest)	N/A	Take this day to allow your body to absorb the training from the previous week. This day will rejuvenate your body for the training week ahead!
Tu	Aerobic Base Run	4–5 miles	This run is to be performed at a low, aerobic intensity (60–70% of max heart rate), a conversational pace, or 45–60 seconds slower than GMRP. The aerobic base run helps develop a robust aerobic system, increasing your fat-burning capabilities.
W	Aerobic Base Run	4–5 miles	This run is to be performed at a low, aerobic intensity (60–70% of max heart rate), a conversational pace, or 45–60 seconds slower than GMRP. The aerobic base run helps develop a robust aerobic system, increasing your fat-burning capabilities.
Th	Aerobic Base Run, plus 5× Strides (relaxed sprints)	4–5 miles	Perform your easy run of 4–5 miles. Then find a nice stretch of road with solid footing to perform your strides afterward.
F	Off Day/ Cross-Training for 30–45 minutes	N/A	Either take the day off from training or cross-train to further the development of your cardiovascular system. The activity you choose should be nonimpact (biking, swimming, using an elliptical, etc.). Keep the effort aerobic and easy (60–70% of max heart rate).
Sat	Aerobic Base Run	5–6 miles	This run is to be performed at a low, aerobic intensity (60–70% of max heart rate), a conversational pace, or 45–60 seconds slower than GMRP. The aerobic base run helps develop a robust aerobic system, increasing your fat-burning capabilities.
Sun	Aerobic Long Run	8–9 miles	The long run should be performed at an easy effort (60–65% of max heart rate), a conversational pace, or 45–60 seconds slower than GMRP. Remember to bring fluids along and take a sip every 15–25 minutes.
TOTAL WEEKLY MILEAGE		25–30 miles	This is a recovery week, or a reduction week. It's a very easy ninth week of training. The decrease in mileage from Week 8 (32–36 miles) to this week is 16–21%.

WEEK 10

This is one of your biggest training weeks so far, and you have two tough workouts scheduled. Hopefully you rested up, both physically and mentally, last week, and you're feeling fresh and ready to begin building your fitness again.

Your hard workouts this week are very similar to the ones you performed in Week 7, but just with more miles added. Reflect on the paces you ran during Week 7, make a note of them going into each workout this week, and then try to hold that same pace for a couple more reps or a couple more miles.

One of the greatest attributes of elite marathon runners is the fact that they can exude emotional control during the early stages of a race or a workout. It is important to think of yourself as a marathoner, night and day, when you're resting and working out. A marathoner possesses excellent patience and displays good judgment when training. They know when to push and when to back off, which is a feeling that can be both practiced and taught. This training program helps teach you how to be patient. You will practice this during your marathon simulation run on Sunday.

Take stock of your fluid supply. Now's the time, if you haven't already, to start consuming the same drink that will be served to you along the marathon course. This will help you get accustomed to the sugar-electrolytes blend. If you're considering using gels to supplement your calorie intake, then practice with those, too, taking one about every five to six miles.

You should start dialing in your prerace meals (dinner the night before and breakfast the day of), as well. Try something that's high in carbohydrates and easily digestible. It will also be important to eat something with carbs and protein immediately after your harder training sessions this week (30 to 60 minutes). This will help speed up your body's recovery process from workout to workout.

WEEK 10	TYPE OF RUN	MILEAGE	NOTES
M	Off Day (complete rest)	N/A	Take this day to allow your body to absorb the training from the previous week. This day will rejuvenate your body for the training week ahead!
Tu	Aerobic Base Run	4–5 miles	This run is to be performed at a low, aerobic intensity (60–70% of max heart rate), a conversational pace, or 45–60 seconds slower than GMRP. The aerobic base run helps develop a robust aerobic system, increasing your fat-burning capabilities.
W	Aerobic Base Run, plus 5× Strides (relaxed sprints)	5–6 miles	Perform your easy run of 5–6 miles. Then find a nice stretch of road with solid footing to perform your strides afterward.
Th	Warm-Up: 1-mile easy run Main Set: 6 × 800m @ GMRP, with equal recovery Cooldown: 1-mile easy run	5 miles	Start with a 1-mile easy warm-up run, take 5 minutes to stretch, and then start the main set. Take a walking recovery interval after each rep of equal time as your 800m interval (e.g., if 800m = 4:30, then your recovery is 4:30). End with a 1-mile easy cooldown run.
F	Off Day/Cross-Training for 30–45 minutes	N/A	Either take the day off from training or cross-train to further the development of your cardiovascular system. The activity you choose should be nonimpact (biking, swimming, using an elliptical, etc.). Keep the effort aerobic and easy (60–70% of max heart rate).
Sat	Aerobic Base Run	6–7 miles	This run is to be performed at a low, aerobic intensity (60–70% of max heart rate), a conversational pace, or 45–60 seconds slower than GMRP. The aerobic base run helps develop a robust aerobic system, increasing your fat-burning capabilities.
Sun	Marathon Simulation Run: 8 miles at 45–60 seconds slower per mile than GMRP, then 4 miles at GMRP, and 1-mile easy cooldown run	13 miles	Start the first 8 miles at 45–60 seconds slower per mile than GMRP, then run 4 miles at GMRP, and finish with a 1-mile easy cooldown run.
TOTAL WEEKLY MILEAGE		33–36 miles	The increase in mileage from Week 8 (32–36 miles) to this week is 0–3%.

WEEK 11

From Weeks 10 to 11, you'll be safely increasing your total weekly mileage from 9 to 11%. After this week, you'll have run 274 to 322 miles over the course of your training. Now would be a good time to grab a new pair of your favorite running shoes. With eight weeks remaining in your training, you might actually want to consider getting two pairs! Keep in mind that, as of race morning, you should have only about 100 miles on the pair of shoes on your feet. That is just enough to break them in so they're comfy and your feet are used to them, but not too much to break down the support or structure of the shoe.

Your long run is really inching up there now, with a 14- to 15-mile run slated for Sunday. It's time to take into consideration the route you're going to run, the time of day, and how hot (or cold) it's going to be while you're out there. You should really try to start simulating what your marathon day might look like. If the course is hilly, then incorporate some undulations into your long run. If the race is at 6:30 a.m., then start your long runs at this time. Think of your Sunday runs as a dress rehearsal for the marathon, minus the enormous crowds.

You are now in what I call the "meat and potatoes" part of your marathon training, just over halfway there. You're now running some serious weekly mileage with long runs that take at least two hours. This is when the calloused physical effect, a general malaise, or an overall tiredness can start to creep in, yet you will still be able to find a way to get in all the mileage and paces required.

It will be interesting to note how much water you're sweating out each hard session. If you know approximately what that number is, then you can make sure you're consuming enough fluids while you're running to offset the loss by a couple of pounds. To figure it out, weigh yourself before and after each long run (see page 29 for the formula).

WEEK 11	TYPE OF RUN	MILEAGE	NOTES
M	Off Day (complete rest)	N/A	Take this day to allow your body to absorb the training from the previous week. This day will rejuvenate your body for the training week ahead!
Tu	Aerobic Base Run	5–6 miles	This run is to be performed at a low, aerobic intensity (60–70% of max heart rate), a conversational pace, or 45–60 seconds slower than GMRP. The aerobic base run helps develop a robust aerobic system, increasing your fat-burning capabilities.
W	Aerobic Base Run, plus 5× Strides (relaxed sprints)	5–6 miles	Perform your easy run of 5–6 miles. Then find a nice stretch of road with solid footing to perform your strides afterward.
Th	Warm-Up: 1-mile easy run Main Set: 6 miles at GMRP Cooldown: 1-mile easy run	8 miles	Start with a 1-mile easy warm-up run, take 5 minutes to stretch, then start the main set. Run 6 miles at GMRP. End with a 1-mile easy cooldown run.
F	Off Day/ Cross-Training for 30–45 minutes	N/A	Either take the day off from training or cross-train to further the development of your cardiovascular system. The activity you choose should be nonimpact (biking, swimming, using an elliptical, etc.). Keep the effort aerobic and easy (60–70% of max heart rate).
Sat	Aerobic Base Run	4–5 miles	This run is to be performed at a low, aerobic intensity (60–70% of max heart rate), a conversational pace, or 45–60 seconds slower than GMRP. The aerobic base run helps develop a robust aerobic system, increasing your fat-burning capabilities.
Sun	Aerobic Long Run	14–15 miles	The long run should be performed at an easy effort (60–65% of max heart rate), a conversational pace, or 45–60 seconds slower than GMRP. Remember to bring fluids along and take a sip every 15–25 minutes.
TOTAL WEEKLY MILEAGE		36–40 miles	The increase in mileage from Week 10 (33–36 miles) to this week is 9–11%.

WEEK 12

Another chance to back off . . . You have a reduction week ahead! These pre-built reduction weeks are here to keep you healthy and allow you to rest in between the hardest weeks.

Use this week to work on strengthening your mental game while your body rests.

During the strides on Thursday, after you've completed your easy aerobic base run, home in on your form. If you have your smartphone with you, set it up on the ground so that you can take a video of yourself doing strides. Make sure you get a side profile. This feedback can be valuable in helping you to refine your mechanics. When athletes see themselves running, and can analyze their arm actions and leg movements, it tends to give them a sense of ownership over their running. Also, these short videos can be displayed on social media, for all your fans to see. Show them you've been training and that you're looking good!

What to look for in the video: If you're displaying excessive bouncing, the angle of your elbows, and where your head is in relation to your shoulders. Revisit chapter 4 for a refresher on running form and mechanics.

WEEK 12	TYPE OF RUN	MILEAGE	NOTES
M	Off Day (complete rest)	N/A	Take this day to allow your body to absorb the training from the previous week. This day will rejuvenate your body for the training week ahead!
Tu	Aerobic Base Run	4–5 miles	This run is to be performed at a low, aerobic intensity (60–70% of max heart rate), a conversational pace, or 45–60 seconds slower than GMRP. The aerobic base run helps develop a robust aerobic system, increasing your fat-burning capabilities.
W	Aerobic Base Run	4–5 miles	This run is to be performed at a low, aerobic intensity (60–70% of max heart rate), a conversational pace, or 45–60 seconds slower than GMRP. The Aerobic Base Run helps develop a more robust aerobic system, increasing your fat-burning capabilities.
Th	Aerobic Base Run, plus 5× Strides (relaxed sprints)	5–6 miles	Perform your easy run of 5–6 miles. Then find a nice stretch of road with solid footing to perform your strides afterward.
F	Off Day/ Cross-Training for 30–45 minutes	N/A	Either take the day off from training or cross-train to further the development of your cardiovascular system. The activity you choose should be nonimpact (biking, swimming, using an elliptical, etc.). Keep the effort aerobic and easy (60–70% of max heart rate).
Sat	Aerobic Base Run	5–6 miles	This run is to be performed at a low, aerobic intensity (60–70% of max heart rate), a conversational pace, or 45–60 seconds slower than GMRP. The aerobic base run helps develop a robust aerobic system, increasing your fat-burning capabilities.
Sun	Aerobic Long Run	9–10 miles	The long run should be performed at an easy effort (60–65% of max heart rate), a conversational pace, or 45–60 seconds slower than GMRP. Remember to bring fluids along and take a sip every 15–25 minutes.
TOTAL WEEKLY MILEAGE		27–32 miles	The decrease in mileage from Week 11 (36–40 miles) to this week is 20–25%.

WEEK 13

This week has the same mileage as Week 11, but the difference is that you will be running more reps during your Yasso 800s on Thursday, and your long run is a mile or two longer.

Consistency and repetition are the keys to success. This is why, to be honest, many elite marathoners live very boring lives. They do the same thing every day for weeks and weeks on end. Up at 6 a.m., have breakfast and coffee, training run (10 to 14 miles) at 8 a.m., have brunch, take a one- to two-hour nap, eat a little snack, put the running shoes on again and hit the road for another six to eight miles, eat dinner, and be back in bed by 9 p.m. They push the repeat button, day after day, week after week, and sometimes month after month. The dedication required to be a professional elite runner is mind-blowing, but also super rewarding, if done properly and with passion.

Think positively this week—during your training runs, throughout the day, and before you go to bed in the evening. Repeat a mantra, such as, "I can do this," "I am doing this," "I've got this," or "I am a marathoner." By repeating it over and over again, your subconscious will start to believe it and you will become it.

Continue to stick to your plan of prescribed workouts. There is no room for error during this time, when the mileage is high and challenging, so make every mile count.

I have a half-marathon time trial planned for the end of Week 14. Begin to think about where you might want to perform such a workout. The course should be like your upcoming marathon race course. If you need to, drive your car around to measure out the route, taking into consideration traffic, terrain, and safety.

WEEK 13	TYPE OF RUN	MILEAGE	NOTES
M	Off Day (complete rest)	N/A	Take this day to allow your body to absorb the training from the previous week. This day will rejuvenate your body for the training week ahead!
Tu	Aerobic Base Run	5–6 miles	This run is to be performed at a low, aerobic intensity (60–70% of max heart rate), a conversational pace, or 45–60 seconds slower than GMRP. The aerobic base run helps develop a robust aerobic system, increasing your fat-burning capabilities.
W	Aerobic Base Run, plus 5× Strides (relaxed sprints)	5–6 miles	Perform your easy run of 5–6 miles. Then find a nice stretch of road with solid footing to perform your strides afterward.
Th	Warm-Up: 1-mile easy run Main Set: 8 × 800m @ GMRP, with equal recovery Cooldown: 1-mile easy run	6 miles	Start with a 1-mile easy warm-up run, take 5 minutes to stretch, and then start the main set. Take a walking recovery interval after each rep of equal time as your 800m interval (e.g., if 800m = 4:30, then your recovery is 4:30). End with a 1-mile easy cooldown run.
F	Off Day/ Cross-Training for 30–45 minutes	N/A	Either take the day off from training or cross-train to further the development of your cardiovascular system. The activity you choose should be nonimpact (biking, swimming, using an elliptical, etc.). Keep the effort aerobic and easy (60–70% of max heart rate).
Sat	Aerobic Base Run	5–6 miles	This run is to be performed at a low, aerobic intensity (60–70% of max heart rate), a conversational pace, or 45–60 seconds slower than GMRP. The aerobic base run helps develop a robust aerobic system, increasing your fat-burning capabilities.
Sun	Aerobic Long Run	15–16 miles	The long run should be performed at an easy effort (60–65% of max heart rate), a conversational pace, or 45–60 seconds slower than GMRP. Remember to bring fluids along and take a sip every 15–25 minutes.
TOTAL WEEKLY MILEAGE		36–40 miles	The increase in mileage from Week 11 (36–40 miles) to this week is 0%.

WEEK 14

Race simulation week is here! This week is an exact replica of your marathon race week, week 20 of your program. This is your opportunity to put all of your training and race logistics to the test.

Treat this week as if you were about to race the marathon. Get your race gear set in the days leading up to the time trial. Have your course picked out. Focus on eating at the same time you would the night before your race and the morning of. Get up early, at least two hours before you start your run, and eat the same meal that you would before the marathon.

Be sure to allow for proper hydration during the time trial. This is when you recruit family and friends to help. Have someone ride a bike next to you for encouragement and moral support, while at the same time handing you fluids every 20 to 25 minutes.

What should your pace for the time trial be? Well, the first half of the run should be comfortable, but then you'll need to push your pace for the second half and finish strong. Remember, you want your fastest time possible for the half-marathon distance to get an accurate gauge of your fitness and what your GMRP should be. Don't worry about pushing too hard and not recovering for next week's workouts—I have taken the liberty of giving you a recovery week. This should leave your legs fresh for the longest run thus far next week.

Your half-marathon time will tell you a lot about your fitness and help you gauge your target goal for marathon race day. Refer to chapter 4 for the formula to determine your marathon pace. Hint: You basically just double it and add 10 to 15 minutes.

WEEK 14	TYPE OF RUN	MILEAGE	NOTES
M	Off Day (complete rest)	N/A	Take this day to allow your body to absorb the training from the previous week. This day will rejuvenate your body for the training week ahead!
Tu	Aerobic Base Run	5–6 miles	This run is to be performed at a low, aerobic intensity (60–70% of max heart rate), a conversational pace, or 45–60 seconds slower than GMRP. The aerobic base run helps develop a robust aerobic system, increasing your fat-burning capabilities.
W	Aerobic Base Run	3–4 miles	This run is to be performed at a low, aerobic intensity (60–70% of max heart rate), a conversational pace, or 45–60 seconds slower than GMRP. The aerobic base run helps develop a robust aerobic system, increasing your fat-burning capabilities.
Th	Aerobic Base Run, plus 5× Strides (relaxed sprints)	5–6 miles	Perform your easy run of 5–6 miles. Then find a nice stretch of road with solid footing to perform your strides afterward.
F	Off Day/ Cross-Training for 30–45 minutes.	N/A	Either take the day off from training or cross-train to further the development of your cardiovascular system. The activity you choose should be nonimpact (biking, swimming, using an elliptical, etc.). Keep the effort aerobic and easy (60–70% of max heart rate).
Sat	Aerobic Base Run, plus 5× Strides (relaxed sprints)	3–4 miles	Perform your easy run of 3–4 miles. Then find a nice stretch of road with solid footing to perform your strides afterward.
Sun	Warm-up: 1-mile easy run Half-marathon time trial, and 1-mile easy run	15 miles	A half-marathon time trial is used as a fitness indicator. Mark a course with your car or Google Earth or use a GPS watch to measure as close to an exact course as possible. Or, if you can, participate in a half-marathon race.
TOTAL WEEKLY MILEAGE		31–35 miles	This is your race simulation week, with a hard half-marathon effort. You're looking for a good performance to base the pace of the marathon. The decrease in mileage from Week 13 (36–40 miles) to this week is 12–13%.

WEEK 15

This week can be considered a reduction week, but that's obviously due to the half-marathon time trial you're just coming off of. You will, however, run the farthest distance of your training program thus far, 15 to 16 miles, this weekend.

Your first few days of training this week might be kind of rocky, as you are coming off of a hard half-marathon effort. You might feel a little more tired than previous Mondays or Tuesdays. Your body may take a few days to recover from a challenging 13.1-mile run, so listen closely to any aches or pains you experience when starting back up.

You deserve a massage this week. If you can't make it in somewhere for one, then simply rub your own legs. Seriously. This was something that I would do after training in college. I didn't have any money to spend on massages, and in fact,

I also gave massages to my teammates for $5 a pop. Remember that the foam roller (and Stick) is your friend.

Another quick recovery tip is to prop your legs up on the wall every now and then, preferably at night, to let them drain out a bit. Draining your legs doesn't break up scar tissue or adhesions, but it does use gravity to help recycle the biological waste products you've accumulated over the last few days of training.

As I mentioned last week, recruiting friends and family to help with your training can make a huge difference, especially during this weekend's long run. If you're training for a 4:30 marathon, which is about a 10:15 per mile pace, and my instructions are to run 45 to 60 seconds slower per mile during the long runs each week, then you should commit to running for about 3 hours (16 miles) on Sunday. You're going to need someone out there to provide moral support and aid. Don't be shy; ask a friend to help you out!

WEEK 15	TYPE OF RUN	MILEAGE	NOTES
M	Off Day (complete rest)	N/A	Take this day to allow your body to absorb the training from the previous week. This day will rejuvenate your body for the training week ahead!
Tu	Aerobic Base Run	4–5 miles	This run is to be performed at a low, aerobic intensity (60–70% of max heart rate), a conversational pace, or 45–60 seconds slower than GMRP. The aerobic base run helps develop a robust aerobic system, increasing your fat-burning capabilities.
W	Aerobic Base Run	4–5 miles	This run is to be performed at a low, aerobic intensity (60–70% of max heart rate), a conversational pace, or 45–60 seconds slower than GMRP. The aerobic base run helps develop a robust aerobic system, increasing your fat-burning capabilities.
Th	Aerobic Base Run, plus 5× Strides (relaxed sprints)	5–6 miles	Perform your easy run of 5–6 miles. Then find a nice stretch of road with solid footing to perform your strides afterward.
F	Off Day/ Cross-Training for 30–45 minutes	N/A	Either take the day off from training or cross-train to further the development of your cardiovascular system. The activity you choose should be nonimpact (biking, swimming, using an elliptical, etc.). Keep the effort aerobic and easy (60–70% of max heart rate).
Sat	Aerobic Base Run	5–6 miles	This run is to be performed at a low, aerobic intensity (60–70% of max heart rate), a conversational pace, or 45–60 seconds slower than GMRP. The aerobic base run helps develop a robust aerobic system, increasing your fat-burning capabilities
Sun	Aerobic Long Run	15–16 miles	The long run should be performed at an easy effort (60–65% of max heart rate), a conversational pace, or 45–60 seconds slower than GMRP. Remember to bring fluids along and take a sip every 15–25 minutes.
TOTAL WEEKLY MILEAGE		33–38 miles	The increase in mileage from Week 14 (31–35 miles) to this week is 6–8%.

WEEK 16

Your biggest week of the season! The next two weeks of big volume are when your marathon toughness and strength are made. It took 15 weeks to build you up to be strong enough to tackle this kind of a training week. Keep your approach the same—run very easy and slowly on the aerobic base run days.

Thursday's Yasso 800s workout is five miles at a high intensity. Be sure to drink your carbohydrate-electrolyte race drink intermittently throughout the workout. This will be especially important in speeding up your recovery before you run 17 to 18 miles at the end of the week.

Sleep is so important right now! Do your best to slip into bed 30 to 60 minutes earlier than usual. I find that reading a book just prior to sleeping helps me pass out a little easier and faster.

Take note of your caffeine and an alcohol consumption. They should be at their lowest during this time. Both will dehydrate you and disturb your sleep patterns, so even if you're tired, try to steer clear of that Americano at 2 p.m.

Sunday is your longest run to date. Congratulations! Remember to just put one foot in front of the other and get it done. Midway through the run, try to reflect on the goals you set out to accomplish. Stay motivated; stay focused on the task at hand. Enjoy the work, and enjoy the fact that you are probably the fittest you have ever been in your life, at least aerobically.

Remember to keep yourself well fueled. You can basically eat whatever you want after a 17- to 18-mile training session. I usually go on a "see-food" diet immediately following a three-plus-hour training run. I see food; I eat it. Enjoy!

WEEK 16	TYPE OF RUN	MILEAGE	NOTES
M	Off Day (complete rest)	N/A	Take this day to allow your body to absorb the training from the previous week. This day will rejuvenate your body for the training week ahead!
Tu	Aerobic Base Run	5–6 miles	This run is to be performed at a low, aerobic intensity (60–70% of max heart rate), a conversational pace, or 45–60 seconds slower than GMRP. The aerobic base run helps develop a robust aerobic system, increasing your fat-burning capabilities.
W	Aerobic Base Run, plus 5× Strides (relaxed sprints)	5–6 miles	Perform your easy run of 5–6 miles. Then find a nice stretch of road with solid footing to perform your strides afterward.
Th	Warm-Up: 1-mile easy run Main Set: 10 × 800m @ GMRP, with equal recovery Cooldown: 1-mile easy run	7 miles	Start with a 1-mile easy warm-up run, take 5 minutes to stretch, and then start the main set. Take a walking recovery interval after each rep of equal time as your 800m interval (e.g., if 800m = 4:30, then your recovery is 4:30). End with a 1-mile easy cooldown run.
F	Off Day/ Cross-Training for 30–45 minutes	N/A	Either take the day off from training or cross-train to further the development of your cardiovascular system. The activity you choose should be nonimpact (biking, swimming, using an elliptical, etc.). Keep the effort aerobic and easy (60–70% of max heart rate).
Sat	Aerobic Base Run	5–6 miles	This run is to be performed at a low, aerobic intensity (60–70% of max heart rate), a conversational pace, or 45–60 seconds slower than GMRP. The aerobic base run helps develop a robust aerobic system, increasing your fat-burning capabilities.
Sun	Aerobic Long Run	17–18 miles	The long run should be performed at an easy effort (60–65% of max heart rate), a conversational pace, or 45–60 seconds slower than GMRP. Remember to bring fluids along and take a sip every 15–25 minutes.
TOTAL WEEKLY MILEAGE		39–43 miles	The increase in mileage from the last big week, Week 13 (36–40 miles), to this week is 7–8%.

WEEK 17

This is your peak week for training volume. You don't need to do anything differently, though, as it's essentially just more of the same.

Take a methodical approach to each day, log one mile at a time, and put one foot in front of the other. It might be time to break out the iPod and listen to some music during your Thursday and Sunday training runs. If you have been listening to music, try mixing it up a little: Add some new songs or download a few podcasts so you can learn along the way.

Carry a water bottle around with you at all times. You need to be nursing 32 to 48 ounces throughout the day, as you are sweating so much during training, even during the winter months.

If you are shooting for a goal time of under four hours in the marathon, then you will need to go the full 20-mile distance at roughly a 10:00-per-mile pace. This adds up to a 3:20 long run. If you are shooting for a time around the five-hour mark for the marathon, then run the shorter 18-mile recommendation, as that will take you just over 3:40.

Don't hesitate to take walk breaks during this long run, if necessary. Try running one to two miles, and then walking for one to two minutes. Use that one to two minutes to consume your drink and energy gels.

WEEK 17	TYPE OF RUN	MILEAGE	NOTES
M	Off Day (complete rest)	N/A	Take this day to allow your body to absorb the training from the previous week. This day will rejuvenate your body for the training week ahead!
Tu	Aerobic Base Run	5–6 miles	This run is to be performed at a low, aerobic intensity (60–70% of max heart rate), a conversational pace, or 45–60 seconds slower than GMRP. The aerobic base run helps develop a robust aerobic system, increasing your fat-burning capabilities.
W	Aerobic Base Run, plus 5× Strides (relaxed sprints)	4–5 miles	Perform your easy run of 4–5 miles. Then find a nice stretch of road with solid footing to perform your strides afterward.
Th	Warm-Up: 1-mile easy run Main Set: 8 miles at GMRP Cooldown: 1-mile easy run	10 miles	Start with a 1-mile easy warm-up run, take 5 minutes to stretch, then start the main set. Run 8 miles at GMRP. End with a 1-mile easy cooldown run.
F	Off Day/ Cross-Training for 30–45 minutes	N/A	Either take the day off from training or cross-train to further the development of your cardiovascular system. The activity you choose should be nonimpact (biking, swimming, using an elliptical, etc.). Keep the effort aerobic and easy (60–70% of max heart rate).
Sat	Aerobic Base Run	5–6 miles	This run is to be performed at a low, aerobic intensity (60–70% of max heart rate), a conversational pace, or 45–60 seconds slower than GMRP. The aerobic base run helps develop a robust aerobic system, increasing your fat-burning capabilities.
Sun	Aerobic Long Run	18–20 miles	The long run should be performed at an easy effort (60–65% of max heart rate), a conversational pace, or 45–60 seconds slower than GMRP. Remember to bring fluids along and take a sip every 15–25 minutes.
TOTAL WEEKLY MILEAGE		42–47 miles	The increase in mileage from Week 16 (39–43 miles) to this week is 7–9%.

WEEK 18

This is the start of your taper period. No one really knows how long the taper should last leading up to a marathon; it's kind of a guessing game, and it changes from person to person. But it is undoubtedly an essential part of training, and the longer the marathon buildup, the longer the taper can be.

David Costill, PhD, in his book *Inside Running: Basics of Sports Physiology*, writes, "Attempts to achieve a peak performance at a specific time adds another dimension to the art of coaching the distance runner." This simply means that each runner is different in how they react to the taper period, or the reduction of mileage and intensity in their training. He goes on to say that many runners often feel fatigued during the two to three weeks leading up to a marathon, during the taper phase, the exact opposite of what you would think. He contributes this to the psychological withdrawal runners experience with the reduced training stimulus.

This would be a good time to consider one last massage before race day to help you flush out all the metabolic by-products you've been producing for the past few months.

All the hard training is now behind you, but it's not time to congratulate yourself just yet. There are some finishing touches that need to be put onto your marathon fitness. Continuing to dial in on your GMRP is very important during these next few weeks.

Thursday's Yasso 800s need to be performed at the same pace you've been running them all season long—stick and commit to those paces. As far as the marathon simulation run is concerned, it is just another dress rehearsal for your marathon. Start off slowly for the first eight miles, and hone your GMRP until you hit the 12-mile mark of the run.

WEEK 18	TYPE OF RUN	MILEAGE	NOTES
M	Off Day (complete rest)	N/A	Take this day to allow your body to absorb the training from the previous week. This day will rejuvenate your body for the training week ahead!
Tu	Aerobic Base Run	4–5 miles	This run is to be performed at a low, aerobic intensity (60–70% of max heart rate), a conversational pace, or 45–60 seconds slower than GMRP. The aerobic base run helps develop a robust aerobic system, increasing your fat-burning capabilities.
W	Aerobic Base Run, plus 5× Strides (relaxed sprints)	5–6 miles	Perform your easy run of 5–6 miles. Then find a nice stretch of road with solid footing to perform your strides afterward.
Th	Warm-Up: 1-mile easy run Main Set: 6 × 800m @ GMRP, with equal recovery Cooldown: 1-mile easy run	5 miles	Start with a 1-mile easy warm-up run, take 5 minutes to stretch, and then start the main set. Take a walking recovery interval after each rep of equal time as your 800m interval (e.g., if 800m = 4:30, then your recovery is 4:30). End with a 1-mile easy cooldown run.
F	Off Day/Cross-Training for 30–45 minutes	N/A	Either take the day off from training or cross-train to further the development of your cardiovascular system. The activity you choose should be non-impact (biking, swimming, using an elliptical, etc.). Keep the effort aerobic and easy (60–70% of max heart rate).
Sat	Aerobic Base Run	5–6 miles	This run is to be performed at a low, aerobic intensity (60–70% of max heart rate), a conversational pace, or 45–60 seconds slower than GMRP.
Sun	Marathon Simulation Run: 8 miles at 45–60 seconds slower per mile than GMRP, then 4 miles at GMRP, and 1-mile easy cooldown run	13 miles	Start the first 8 miles at 45–60 seconds slower per mile than GMRP, then run 4 miles at GMRP, and finish with a 1-mile easy cooldown run.
TOTAL WEEKLY MILEAGE		32–35 miles	The decrease in mileage from Week 17 (42–47 miles, your peak week) to this week is 23–25%.

WEEK 19

The penultimate week before your marathon! This week will decrease in mileage by about 12% from last week, keeping with the theme of resting your body.

The way my college coach explained the taper phase to me was that our bodies are in a state of depletion all during the season leading up to the peak race. Then, once the volume and intensity levels are decreased, our bodies are allowed to catch back up and rebuild, which means we can get stronger because of the rest. He called this physiological phenomenon "super-compensation." We go from a chronically fatigued state to stronger than before. This, ultimately, is the desired adaptive response to a training stimulus.

Your two workouts this week are ones that you've done before, and they should be performed at the same paces you've been training at throughout your training plan. You don't need to do anything fancy this week; just go through the motions and put in the work as set forth in the plan.

This week, during each of your training runs, remember to save a little something for race day. As your mileage and intensity are reduced, you will begin to feel energized and you'll probably be tempted to run your workouts faster than you should. This is when you will need to exude emotional control and self-govern your output. Hold back now, and you'll be thankful you did come race day!

WEEK 19	TYPE OF RUN	MILEAGE	NOTES
M	Off Day (complete rest)	N/A	Take this day to allow your body to absorb the training from the previous week. This day will rejuvenate your body for the training week ahead!
Tu	Aerobic Base Run	4–5 miles	This run is to be performed at a low, aerobic intensity (60–70% of max heart rate), a conversational pace, or 45–60 seconds slower than GMRP. The aerobic base run helps develop a robust aerobic system, increasing your fat-burning capabilities.
W	Aerobic Base Run, plus 5× Strides (relaxed sprints)	4–5 miles	Perform your easy run of 4–5 miles. Then find a nice stretch of road with solid footing to perform your strides afterward.
Th	Warm-Up: 1-mile easy run Main Set: 4 × 800m @ GMRP, with equal recovery Cooldown: 1-mile easy run	6 miles	Start with a 1-mile easy warm-up run, take 5 minutes to stretch, and then start the main set. Run 1 mile at your GMRP, and take a 3:00 recovery between each mile repeat. End with a 1-mile easy cooldown run.
F	Off Day/Cross-Training for 30–45 minutes	N/A	Either take the day off from training or cross-train to further the development of your cardiovascular system. The activity you choose should be non-impact (biking, swimming, using an elliptical, etc.). Keep the effort aerobic and easy (60–70% of max heart rate).
Sat	Aerobic Base Run	4–5 miles	This run is to be performed at a low, aerobic intensity (60–70% of max heart rate), a conversational pace, or 45–60 seconds slower than GMRP. The aerobic base run helps develop a robust aerobic system, increasing your fat-burning capabilities.
Sun	Marathon Simulation Run: 4 miles at 45–60 seconds slower per mile than GMRP, then 4 miles at GMRP, and 1-mile easy cooldown run	9 miles	Start the first 4 miles at 45–60 seconds slower per mile than GMRP, then run 4 miles at GMRP, and finish with a 1-mile easy cooldown run.
TOTAL WEEKLY MILEAGE		27–30 miles	The decrease in mileage from Week 18 (31–34 miles) to this week is 11–12%.

WEEK 20

Race week is here! Remember, you have done this before. Think back to Week 14 and your half-marathon time trial—you've rehearsed this. Even if the rehearsal didn't go well, at least you now have an idea of how you can correct it for a more successful race.

The theme from last week, save a little something for race day, applies to this week, too. Keep the miles easy, even though it might be tempting to fly through some of your runs. You need to hold back the best you can.

Keep your nutrition and hydration in mind all week long as well. Most marathoners gain weight during the last 10 days or so of the taper. They are so used to eating copious amounts of food during the heavy weeks of training that it becomes a habit. Believe it or not, this is a desired weight gain. I repeat, this is a desired weight gain. Most of the weight that is being added during the taper is water weight, along with muscle glycogen that's being stored up for race day. The average runner will gain anywhere from two to four pounds in the final week and a half of training, which is weight that is needed for making that long journey from start to finish.

Get off your feet this week as much as possible. Prop your legs up at night, or better yet, elevate them to drain any residual fluid retention. Stay relaxed. Read a book, have fun with friends. I find that laughter is great during the days leading up to any race, so rent a funny movie.

Rest easy knowing you have done all the work necessary to execute a great race. Reflect on your training by looking through your logbook and take note of all the running you have done this season. Hint: It's been a lot! Up until this week, you've run between 541 and 622 miles. That's about the distance from Los Angeles to Salt Lake City!

With all the advice, instructions, and tips you've acquired over the last 20 weeks, all that's left for you to do is to simply get out there and race. Enjoy the tail end of this journey—it's your final act!

WEEK 20	TYPE OF RUN	MILEAGE	NOTES
M	Off Day (complete rest)	N/A	Take this day to allow your body to absorb the training from the previous week. This day will rejuvenate your body for the training week ahead!
Tu	Aerobic Base Run	5–6 miles	This run is to be performed at a low, aerobic intensity (60–70% of max heart rate), a conversational pace, or 45–60 seconds slower than GMRP. The aerobic base run helps develop a robust aerobic system, increasing your fat-burning capabilities.
W	Aerobic Base Run	3–4 miles	This run is to be performed at a low, aerobic intensity (60–70% of max heart rate), a conversational pace, or 45–60 seconds slower than GMRP. The aerobic base run helps develop a robust aerobic system, increasing your fat-burning capabilities.
Th	Aerobic Base Run, plus 5× Strides (relaxed sprints)	5–6 miles	Perform your easy run of 5–6 miles. Then find a nice stretch of road with solid footing to perform your strides afterward.
F	Off Day/ Cross-Training for 30–45 minutes	N/A	Either take the day off from training or cross-train to further the development of your cardiovascular system. The activity you choose should be nonimpact (biking, swimming, using an elliptical, etc.). Keep the effort aerobic and easy (60–70% of max heart rate).
Sat	Aerobic Base Run, plus 5× Strides (relaxed sprints)	3–4 miles	Perform your easy run of 3–4 miles. Then find a nice stretch of road with solid footing to perform your strides afterward.
Sun	Marathon Race	26.2M	Have a great race! Enjoy.
TOTAL WEEKLY MILEAGE		42.2–46.2 miles	Race week! Stick to your racing plan!

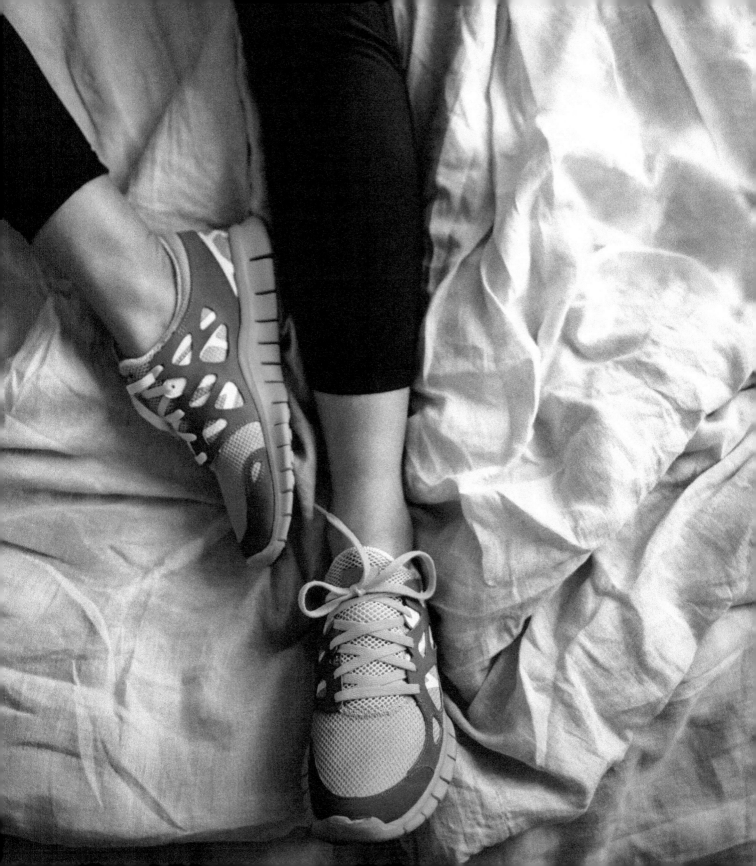

9

BEFORE THE RACE

In the final days and hours leading up to your marathon, it's important for you to reflect on your training and realize that this is the moment when your preparation—all of those miles and early mornings—comes together. I always tell my pro and age-group athletes to take a deep breath, control their excitement and fear, and then channel that into a great performance, a performance that they (and their friends and family) will be extremely proud of. And remember to keep it all in perspective—there will inevitably be other first-time marathoners out there with you, and they will be just as nervous as (if not more than) you, because chances are they didn't follow a training plan that prepped them quite as well for the 26.2-mile journey as yours did.

This chapter will cover your final checklist for race day, including a list of dos and don'ts, plus things that you will need to remember to bring with you on marathon morning. You've been training for the last 20 weeks for this very moment—it's important to not let one little item on your checklist slip through the cracks and negatively impact your race.

10 THINGS TO DO BEFORE RACE DAY

1. NOTHING NEW! This is the golden rule you need to follow on the days leading up to your marathon: Don't try anything new. You should eat only familiar foods, drink only familiar beverages, and wear only familiar gear (shirts, shorts, sports bras, socks, shoes, etc.) on race day. In other words, if you haven't tried it in training, then don't try it now. Many runners are tempted to experiment with new gadgets, gels, or other running products they find at the race expo the day before the race, but now is not the time for experimentation. Do what you already know works. And if you see something you like at the expo, buy it, and then try it in the training leading up to your next race.

2. PRACTICE WHAT YOU ARE GOING TO EAT IN THE DAYS (AND WEEKS) LEADING UP TO YOUR RACE. You should be experimenting with a prerace meal that is high in complex carbohydrates and passes through your digestive system easily. It is also wise to eat dinner early (4 or 5 p.m.) the night before a long run or race. If you're traveling to your race, then about three to four weeks out start looking for a restaurant nearby that serves the prerace meal of your choice and make a reservation. The prerace meal is always a bit easier if you're at home the night before.

3. ABSTAIN FROM ALCOHOL AND COFFEE IN THE FINAL DAYS LEADING UP TO YOUR RACE. I always advise athletes to do this, with a goal of keeping your body as hydrated as possible. Of course, coffee the morning of the race is not a bad idea, but only if that's part of your normal long-run routine. One reason I tell folks to back off on their coffee consumption in the days leading up to a marathon is that during that final week, you're running very little in order to rest your legs, and the lower training volume could adversely affect your typical sleeping pattern. Athletes tend to be cranky and restless during the taper phase due to the extra energy being built up, too.

4. GET YOUR SLEEP! Your goal for race week is to rest as much as possible. I once knew an Olympic Race Walking coach who would tell his athletes, "If you don't have bedsores on your body, then you aren't resting enough." Kick your feet up frequently and sleep as much as you can in the final days leading up to your race.

5. STUDY THE COURSE MAP. You may have reviewed it before you signed up for the race, just to make sure you weren't running up Mount Everest at the 20-mile mark or anything, but it's a good idea to refresh your map memory during the week of your marathon. Look for where the aid stations are and note their frequency (every mile, every three miles, etc.). Look at how the staging corrals are set up so you know where to go in the morning and where the porta potties will be. Usually race directors send an email out with final race-day instructions, so be sure to read that closely.

6. PLAN FOR A FAMILY REUNION AFTER THE RACE. Many races have a designated "family reunion" area to help you locate your loved ones after you cross the finish line. Be sure to identify this on your course map and let your friends and family members know where to go. Also, give them your estimated pace/finish time to help make it easier for them to follow you on the course and possibly see you cross that line in the end. You don't want to miss any prime photo-ops! Many bigger marathons have a race-day athlete tracker app that can be downloaded onto supporters' smartphones, too.

7. TRIM YOUR TOENAILS. Seriously. Sometimes it's the smallest things that can cause the biggest amount of pain and suffering during your race. Remember that your feet will swell and lengthen over the course of those 26.2 miles. The last thing you want is your toenails getting jammed up in the front of your shoes at mile 16!

8. CHECK THE LOCAL FORECAST. This is particularly important. Just because you were planning to run your marathon at a certain temperature doesn't mean it will play out that way, and you want to be as prepared as possible. The weather conditions should not only dictate what you wear on race day, but also if you need to adjust your goal race pace. If it's on the hotter side, warmer than what you've been training in, then it would be wise to slow your pace down by 10 to 30 seconds per mile and to consume fluids at a more frequent rate. Check the event's website in the days leading up to your race to see if there are any updates or warnings for participants.

9. PICK YOUR RACE OUTFIT. And then set it out the night before your race so nothing is forgotten in the morning. Remember, you'll want to wear something that you have trained (and performed long runs) consistently in. Consider the weather. And be sure to think about everything you'll need from head to toe, from a hat and socks to a cheap sweatshirt that you can toss after you start the race if it's chilly. The clothing left behind on the course is often donated to charity, so don't feel bad about literally throwing anything away during your run.

10. VISIT THE RACE EXPO AS SOON AS POSSIBLE. You'll most likely have to make your way to the race expo at some point to pick up your bib number. Do this as soon as you arrive in the city you're racing in, and try to make it as quick and painless as possible. As tempting as it is to walk around, visiting all the booths selling the latest and greatest running products, you'll want to save your legs for the race and allow yourself enough time to recover afterward, before the starting gun fires.

10 THINGS TO BRING WITH YOU ON RACE DAY

Aside from the clothes on your back and the socks and shoes on your feet, here's what to bring with you on race day.

1. EXTRA WARM CLOTHES, ALONG WITH YOUR RACING OUTFIT: This will be especially important if the early-morning temps are supposed to be chilly. Athletes want to avoid involuntary shivering just prior to the starting gun. This uncontrollable action burns through precious muscle glycogen in your body that you will need to tap into during your race. Stay warm for as long as possible before you start running and begin to warm up naturally.

2. A WATER BOTTLE AND SNACKS: Sip and graze on these while you wait to start to help keep your blood sugar and hydration up. Bring an electrolyte-replacement drink to help keep everything topped off. It's okay to eat a little granola bar, banana, or bites of a bagel just prior to the race, as long as you've tried it in training and had your normal pre-long-run breakfast as well. Remember, you will be running at a low intensity during the race, and your ability to digest food should be good at this slower pace.

3. A PACE CHEAT SHEET: Bring a pace band, or write your splits (times you should finish each mile) down on your hand to help you maintain a steady goal race pace throughout the marathon. If you're like me and wear a simple stopwatch while you run, then writing down your projected splits on your hand or forearm is important as a way to cross-reference when you pass certain mile markers. If you've been wearing a GPS watch in practice that gives you instant feedback regarding pace, then go ahead and use that device instead.

4. BAND-AIDS: Folks, you're going to want to cover your nipples with these. Chafing hurts everywhere, but when your shirt rubs against your nipples, it can cause bleeding as well, so covering them up with a protective layer is super important.

5. YOUR RACE BIB: Your time will not be recorded, nor will you get any professional race photos, if you're not wearing your race bib/number. Bring extra safety pins to stick the bib on to your shirt, too—even if you don't need them, someone around you might.

6. YOUR PHONE: You'll need it if you want to capture and share the awesomeness of this experience, as most first-time marathoners do. Remember to hashtag the race if you post anything.

7. YOUR RACE BAG: At most bigger marathons, you get a clear bag when you check in. Fill it with whatever you want to have on race morning and won't need during the race (car keys, wallet, phone, headphones, extra clothes, Vaseline, etc.). There should be a place to drop your bag off (it's marked with your bib number) at the start, and then a place to pick it back up at the finish.

8. VASELINE (OR OTHER KIND OF CHAFE-RESISTANT GEL/POWDER): Apply liberally to those pesky chafing areas (under the arms, toes, inner thighs, etc.).

9. A WATCH: Wear it to bed the night before, so that you have one less thing to remember in the morning. The race may have timing clocks on the course at every mile or 5K, but the time being displayed is usually based on when the pros crossed the starting line, not you (and everyone else). You'll need your own device to monitor your own pace/time.

10. SUN PROTECTION: Bring sunscreen, especially if it's going to be sunny. A hat is helpful in both sunny and rainy weather as well. Just be sure it's one that you've worn on some of your long runs already.

10 THINGS YOU DON'T WANT TO FORGET!

1. What starting corral are you in? Line up correctly and follow the instructions provided by the race organization website or volunteers on-site for safety purposes. And no, you are not a herd of cattle, but you might feel like one on race morning.

2. If it's wet or cold outside, be sure to keep your layers on during the early part of the race. You can always shed an old sweatshirt or rain poncho after you warm up a bit.

3. Know where the aid stations are along the course so that you can time your fluid intake appropriately. Your level of thirst will be dictated by the heat index, so be prepared to consume more if it's warmer on race day than it was during most of your long training runs.

4. Be patient when you go through the aid stations. Allow runners ahead of you to get their drinks first, since they were in front of you. And be polite: The aid stations are usually staffed by volunteers who are out there simply to provide support. I always make a point to thank them all for being out there when I run through.

5. Sometimes nature calls! When you gotta go, you gotta go. There's no shame in stopping at a porta potty along the course, if needed. After all, that's what they're there for! And don't rush things—spending an extra minute in there is way better than having to stop again later.

6. Remember to smile. Often. You never know when your face will end up on social media or even in a promotional campaign for the race organization. And, most importantly, remember to smile and raise your hands overhead as you cross the finish line. You just finished a marathon! (And you might want to frame that photo at some point.) *Side note:* All elite runners at the New York City Marathon are instructed the day before the race that if they win, and they're caught stopping their watches at the finish line, then they will not be paid their prize money. To stop their watches, athletes reach across their bibs, which blocks the sponsor's logo. Plus, it makes for a horrible finish line photo.

7. Many marathons are really packed at the starting line, so you might want to consider riding out the first wave of runners and letting the crowd thin out a little bit for those first few miles before you start sprinting past everyone. There's no need for pushing or yelling. Just simply move around folks, and remember others are out there for the same reason as you, to make their way to that almighty marathon finish line.

8. Always remember that there'll be "good miles" and there'll be "rough miles." If you're feeling crummy at mile eight during the race, be patient and know that the next mile or two will likely feel better. This feeling of "good one mile, bad the next" often has to do with how your body is metabolizing carbs and fat while you run—it's working hard to find the optimal combo in the middle stages of the race.

9. Start off conservatively for the first 20 miles of the race. Yes, 20. Stick to your goal race pace that you've been training at. Runners often say that the 20-mile mark is kind of when you feel like you've finished the first half of the race.

10. If something on your body starts to hurt, then focus on something else! Fix your attention on the road ahead or the spectators' encouraging signs (see chapter 7) to help brighten your mood. For example, if your hamstring starts to tighten up, tell it to relax and remind yourself that you have five other hamstrings that are working just fine, and then search for a funny sign.

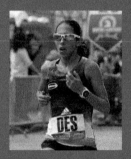

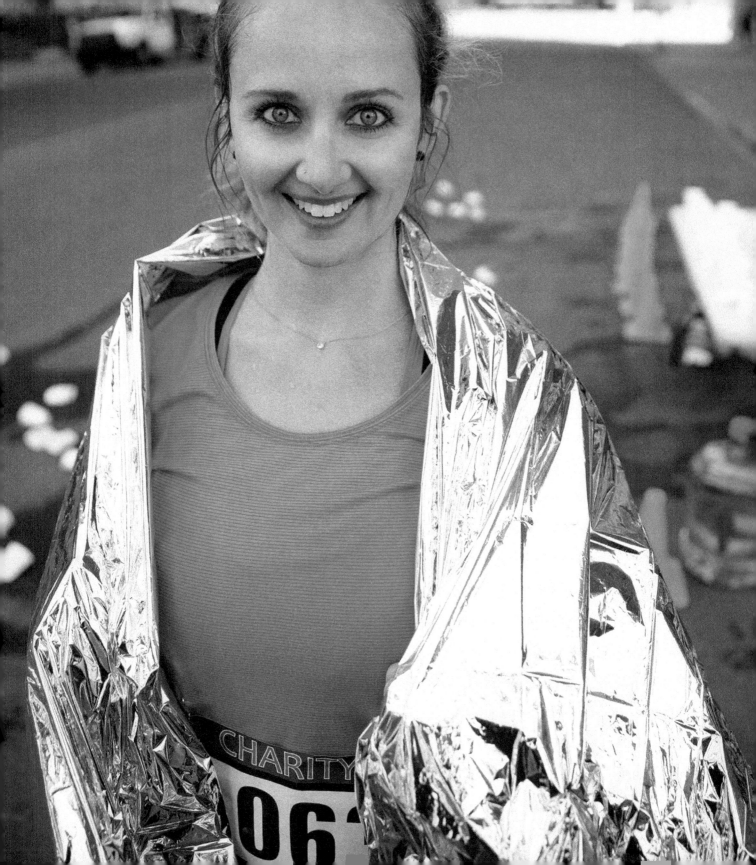

10
AFTER THE RACE

Finishing a marathon is an accomplishment of immense physical and mental strength. You should be very proud of yourself for committing to the program, sticking with it, even when the going got tough, and seeing it all the way through to the finish. *Congratulations! You deserve that medal!*

During your marathon training and the marathon itself, you've given your body a bit of a beating to make it stronger, and now's your chance to recover! Give yourself two to three weeks off, or at least with reduced, low-impact activity. After this recovery period, it will be time for you to reassess your goals for the future. Does another marathon lie ahead? Maybe you'll shoot for a faster time or run a different course? Will you move on to another distance? Take this opportunity to ask yourself, "What challenge is next?"

RECOVERY

I know a few runners who abstain from certain foods and beverages when they're in serious marathon training. This type of discipline makes for a great postrace celebration! Planning an amazing postrace meal with your friends and family gives you something pleasurable to look forward to immediately after you cross that finish line, rather than solely focusing on grinding through all those miles.

Warning: Immediately after the race, your stomach might be churning a bit from all the sugary beverages and snacks you consumed along the route. If that's indeed the case, then eat a small amount of salty or savory food 30 to 60 minutes after the race. Colder marathons often serve soup at the finish, which is easily digestible and usually packed with sodium. Once your appetite returns, it would be great to get in some carbohydrates, like granola, bagels, potatoes, or pasta, and lean protein to help replenish your body's depleted stores.

If you're looking for some recovery strategies after the race, refer to chapter 6 for ideas. Recovering from a marathon is the same as recovering from a long run—it's just that you're probably going to be even more sore after running your *longest run ever* (by six to eight miles!) at a relatively fast pace.

One good rule of thumb on how to recover from your race is to take one day off for every mile run (for a marathon, that means 26 days) to allow your body the opportunity to fully recover from the effort and training. At minimum, I recommend taking two complete weeks off, and then starting back with easy runs (two to four miles) every other day until you hit the 26th day after your race. At that point, you can swing back into your normal routine . . . or start training for something different.

WHAT NEXT?

So what's next, you ask? I encourage you to luxuriate in this incredible sense of accomplishment that you've just earned. Reflect on all the hard work you've put in the last four to five months and the dedication that it took for you to achieve this newfound strength and fitness. Now imagine harnessing that same work ethic and focusing it on another goal. Maybe you want to do another marathon because this one felt too easy (good for you!). Or maybe there's another physical challenge that's been nagging at you for a while, like hiking the Grand Canyon or climbing a mountain. Now that you've reached a supreme level of fitness, the possibilities are endless. And if your future goal involves training for another marathon, or even a half-marathon, be sure to glance back at this training program for reference.

And remember, your next goal doesn't necessarily have to be a physical one. Training for a marathon is a prime example of setting a goal for yourself and then working backward from there to help guide your path to achievement. Replaying the goal in your mind for months and visualizing it coming to fruition can have a huge positive effect on you. This approach can spill over into other aspects of your life as well. You built a good team to help you get to the finish line by recruiting friends and family and surrounding yourself with positive support. You can repeat that process to succeed in other parts of your life—you really just need to be proactive and follow a well-thought-out plan.

ASK A PRO

SHALANE FLANAGAN, FOUR-TIME OLYMPIC MARATHONER AND OLYMPIC SILVER MEDALIST

How do you celebrate a great run?

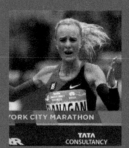

To get through the grueling workouts, 17 miles a day or three-hour-long runs, I not only visualize the finish line and the overwhelming sense of accomplishment . . . I dream of postrace celebrating!

For some marathons, I dream of indulging in an absurd amount of my favorite naughty foods, like doughnuts. My go-to place at home is called Sesame Donuts. I love pastries and usually eat a sampling of them until I'm sick. Other indulgences include local Oregon IPAs and pinot noir, or my favorite, a juicy burger and French fries!

Vacations are also celebratory must-haves for me. They allow me to break from my monk lifestyle of deliberate sleep and eating habits.

After I ran my first NYC marathon, my husband and entire training group took a trip to Maui. It was one of the best trips we've ever taken because I got to celebrate with my best friends.

After I finished the Berlin marathon, a huge plate of fries and a week of road-tripping around Europe with my parents were awaiting me as a celebration.

It is always worth digging deep in the training because I believe it makes the doughnuts taste sweeter!

AFTER THE RACE

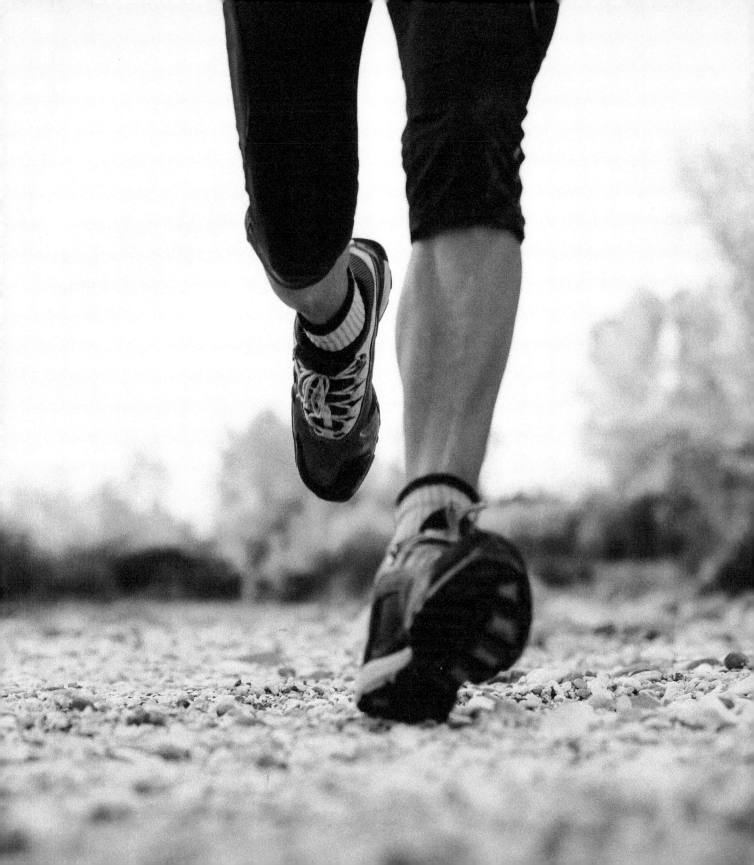

PREDICTING YOUR RACE TIME

1 MILE	5K	10K	10 MILES	½ MAR	MARATHON
6:00	19:57	41:36	1:08:53	1:31:47	3:11:22
6:15	20:47	43:20	1:11:46	1:35:37	3:19:21
6:30	21:37	45:04	1:14:38	1:39:26	3:27:19
6:45	22:27	46:48	1:17:30	1:43:16	3:35:18
7:00	23:17	48:32	1:20:22	1:47:05	3:43:16
7:15	24:07	50:16	1:23:14	1:50:55	3:51:15
7:30	24:56	52:00	1:26:07	1:54:44	3:59:13
7:45	25:46	53:44	1:28:59	1:58:34	4:07:11
8:00	26:36	55:28	1:31:51	2:02:23	4:15:10
8:15	27:26	57:12	1:34:43	2:06:13	4:23:08
8:30	28:16	58:56	1:37:36	2:10:02	4:31:07
8:45	29:06	1:00:40	1:40:28	2:13:51	4:39:05

Continued »

1 MILE	5K	10K	10 MILES	½ MAR	MARATHON
9:00	29:56	1:02:24	1:43:20	2:17:41	4:47:04
9:15	30:46	1:04:08	1:46:12	2:21:30	4:55:02
9:30	31:36	1:05:52	1:49:04	2:25:20	5:03:00
9:45	32:25	1:07:36	1:51:57	2:29:09	5:10:59
10:00	33:15	1:09:20	1:54:49	2:32:59	5:18:57
10:15	34:05	1:11:04	1:57:41	2:36:48	5:26:56
10:30	34:55	1:12:48	2:00:33	2:40:38	5:34:54
10:45	35:45	1:14:32	2:03:26	2:44:27	5:42:53
11:00	36:35	1:16:16	2:06:18	2:48:17	5:50:51
11:15	37:25	1:18:00	2:09:10	2:52:06	5:58:49
11:30	38:15	1:19:44	2:12:02	2:55:56	6:06:48
11:45	39:04	1:21:28	2:14:54	2:59:45	6:14:46
12:00	39:54	1:23:12	2:17:47	3:03:35	6:22:45

Source: www.runnersworld.com/tools/race-time-predictor

RESOURCES

I encourage you to delve a little deeper into some of the resources I used when writing this book. I've written a sentence or two on each resource to help you gain a sense of the information that I gleaned.

CHAPTER 1

BAA.org. This site is useful for finding eligible courses for qualification into the country's oldest and most prestigious marathon, as well as the qualifying-time standards. http://www.baa.org

RunningUSA.org. It was fun and inspiring to learn the stats pertaining to the amount of people running marathons in the United States. http://www.runningUSA.org

Womensrunning.com. This site was essential in finding the world's most popular marathons. http://womensrunning.competitor. com/2017/04/races/22-worlds-most-popular-marathons_74247#4R6sLIfGjjCLcpFW.97.

CHAPTER 2

Dengate, Jeff. "Choose the Right Running Socks." *Runner's World*. Accessed October 8, 2017. http://www.runnersworld.com/running-apparel/choose-the-right-running-socks. This article provides some useful pointers for choosing the best running socks for you.

Humphrey, Luke. *Hansons Half-Marathon Method: Run Your Best Half-Marathon the Hansons Way.* Boulder, CO: VeloPress, 2014. This book was a great resource for its many training ideas and workout suggestions. It's an extremely comprehensive book for all runners.

Jabr, Ferris. "Let's Get Physical: The Psychology of Effective Workout Music." *Scientific American*. Accessed October 8, 2017. http://www.scientificamerican.com/article/psychology-workout-music. Here's a wonderful article illustrating the use of music to enhance the athletic experience.

"Sports Bras: How to Choose." REI.com. Accessed October 8, 2017. http://www.rei.com/learn/expert-advice/sports-bras.html. This website had many top tips for purchasing the perfect running sports bra for women of all shapes and sizes.

CHAPTER 3

Corliss, Julie. "Eating Too Much Refined Sugar Increases the Risk of Dying with Heart Disease." *Harvard Heat Letter*. Accessed October 8, 2017. https://www.health.harvard.edu/blog/eating-too-much-added-sugar-increases-the-risk-of-dying-with-heart-disease-201402067021. We all thought it was cholesterol and red meat!

Eberle, Suzanne Girard, MS, RD. *Endurance Sports Nutrition: Eating Plans for Optimal Training, Racing, and Recovery.* Champaign, Ill.: Human Kinetics Publishers, 2000. If you want to learn more regarding the endurance athlete's diet, please pick up this very comprehensive book.

"Healthy Hydration." The American Council on Exercise. Accessed October 8, 2017. https://www.acefitness.org/fitfacts/pdfs/fitfacts/itemid_2639.pdf. This site provides great recommendations for fluid intake.

Howard, Nancy. "Running Tip: The Importance of Hydration." SparkPeople.com. Accessed October 8, 2017. http://www.sparkpeople.com/blog/blog.asp?post=running_tip_the_importance_of_hydration. This article had some great hydration suggestions and outlined the importance during training.

McDevitt, Kim. "Blueberries Power Performance." RunnersWorld.com. Accessed October 8, 2017. http://www.runnersworld.com/nutrition/blueberries-power-performance. Blueberries are a superfood for endurance athletes, packed full of antioxidants.

RunnersConnect.net. I used this site to calculate caloric intake for runners based on their age (https://runnersconnect.net/training/tools/calorie-calculator). This site is a great resource for runners of all abilities, filled with tips and helpful information.

USDA.gov. The US Department of Agriculture developed the educational guidelines for eating the essential foods over the years. Visit their site at http://www.usda.gov.

Utzschneider, Cathy. *Mastering Running: Run Faster and Stronger While Avoiding Injuries.* Champaign, Ill.: Human Kinetics Publishers, 2014. This is a great read for all-around health and fitness for runners of all ages.

Wang, Xia, Yingying Ouyang, Jun Liu, Minmin Zhu, Gang Zhao, Wei Bao, Frank B Hu. "Fruit and Vegetable Consumption and Mortality from All Causes, Cardiovascular Disease, and Cancer: Systematic Review and Dose-Response Meta-Analysis of Prospective Cohort Studies." *BMJ* 349 (2014). doi:https://doi.org/10.1136/bmj.g4490. This article from *BMJ* outlines the importance of eating fruits and vegetables—a great reminder!

CHAPTER 4

RunnersWorld.com. Thanks for the use of your calculator for determining target heart rate.

CHAPTER 5

Wharton, Jim, and Phil Wharton. *The Whartons' Stretch Book: Featuring the Breakthrough Method of Active-Isolated Stretching.* New York: TimesBooks, 1996. This book provided guidance for the top five stretches for marathon runners.

CHAPTER 6

Keflezighi, Meb, and Scott Douglas. *Meb for Mortals: How to Run, Think, and Eat like a Champion Marathoner.* New York: Rodale, 2015. In his book, Keflezighi, one of America's best marathoners, describes in detail his best cross-training techniques for maintaining his fitness well into his forties.

CHAPTER 8

Costill, David L. *Inside Running: Basics of Sports Physiology.* Carmel, Ind.: Benchmark Press, 1986. As one of the leaders in running physiology, Costill, through his laboratory work, has given valuable training insight to coaches and athletes for decades.
Lydiard, Arthur. *Running to the Top.* Aachen, Germany: Meyer & Meyer Sport, 2012. Lydiard gives a great perspective on training from the golden era of distance running. His philosophies from the 1960s are still used by coaches.

INDEX

ABOUT THE AUTHOR

Andrew Kastor started his running career in the early 1990s, at the age of 14, when he competed in cross-country racing, track, and road racing while attending Fountain Valley High School in Southern California.

He then went on to pursue a degree in Exercise Physiology from Adams State University in Alamosa, Colorado. While in college, Andrew's commitment to the sport of running continued to grow as he competed in cross-country racing and track, specializing in the middle-distance events.

Post-graduation, Andrew moved to Mammoth Lakes, California, where he created and coached a nonprofit running club called the High Sierra Striders. He's now the head coach for the Mammoth Track Club (a professional and adult running club).

Andrew currently resides in Mammoth Lakes with his wife, Deena (Olympic marathon bronze medalist and American record holder in the marathon and half-marathon), and their daughter, Piper Bloom.

ACKNOWLEDGMENTS

I just wanted to take a moment to say thank you! Thank you so much for getting out on the road, for motivating me to write this book, and for including me in your personal journey of running your first marathon. I'm so glad you signed up and stuck with the plan. And I wish you the best of luck with whatever challenge you (inevitably) decide to tackle next.

CPSIA information can be obtained
at www.ICGtesting.com
Printed in the USA
BVHW06s0423280818
525737BV00002B/2/P